Our Mum Bought a MOUNTAIN Bike

Stewart Williams

Contact / follow me on...

Stewart Williams - Author / Illustrator

stewart_williams_author

Stewwriter@outlook.com

Tassie Mountain Bike Trails

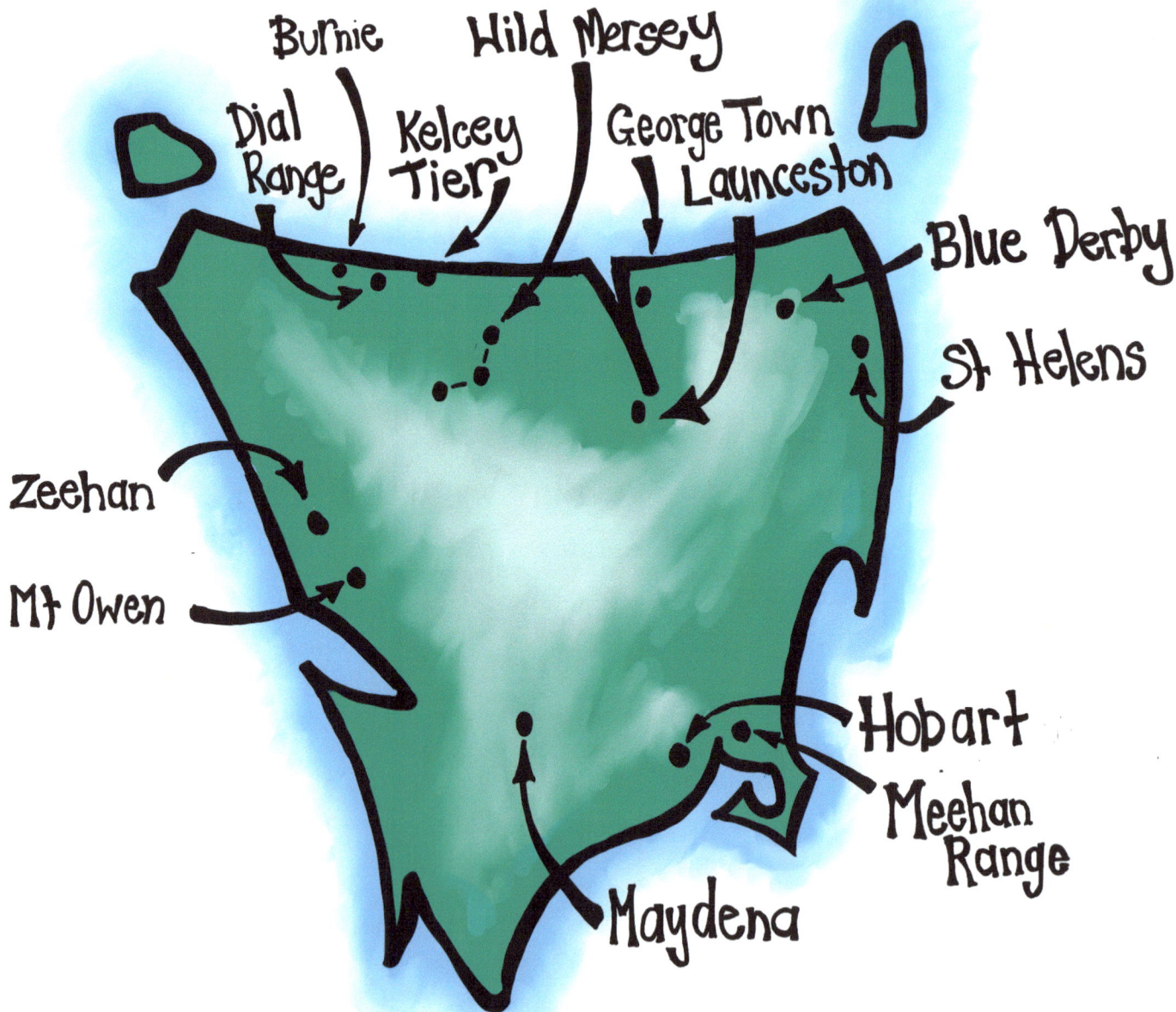

Burnie

Hild Mersey

Dial Range

Kelcey Tier

George Town
Launceston

Blue Derby

St Helens

Zeehan

Mt Owen

Hobart

Meehan Range

Maydena

Our dad bought a mountain bike, and we know how that went.
All the crashes that he had,
all the money that he spent.

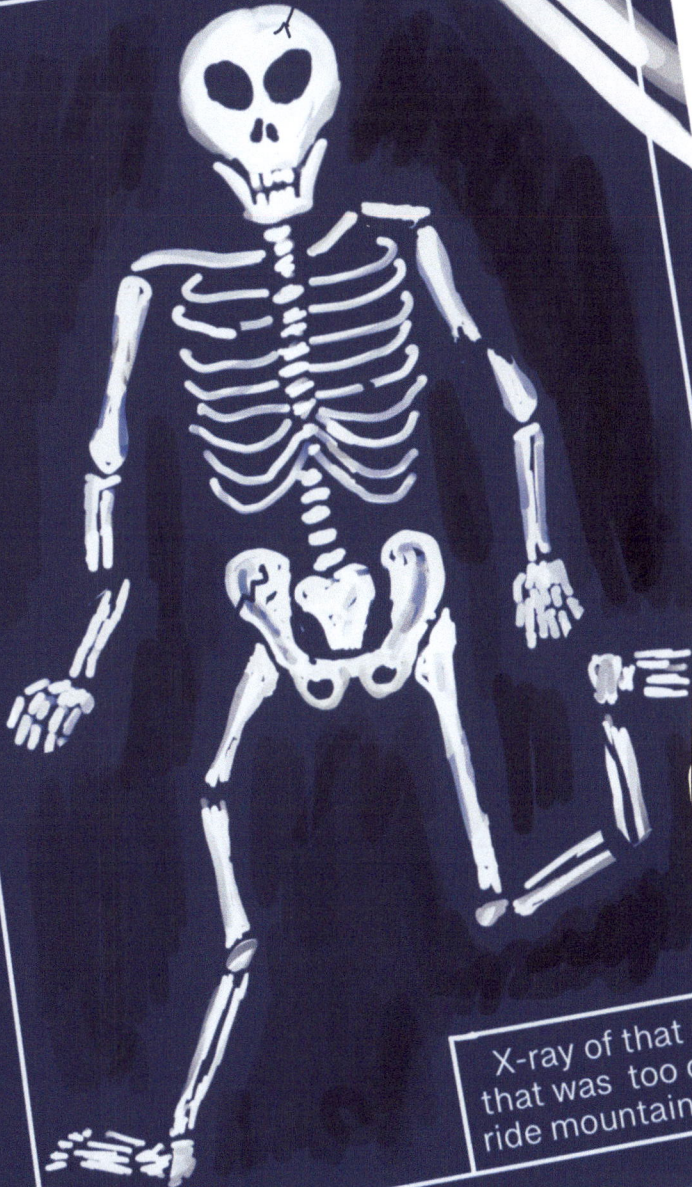

X-ray of that guy that was too old to ride mountain bikes

Bank statement

BB Bank of Biking

Date	Funds
Start of month	Lots of money
Mid month	Not looking good
End of month	Where did all that go?
Total expenditure	Oh dear...

So, we've ridden with Dad
everywhere that he's been.
But Mum never came,
she just wasn't that keen.

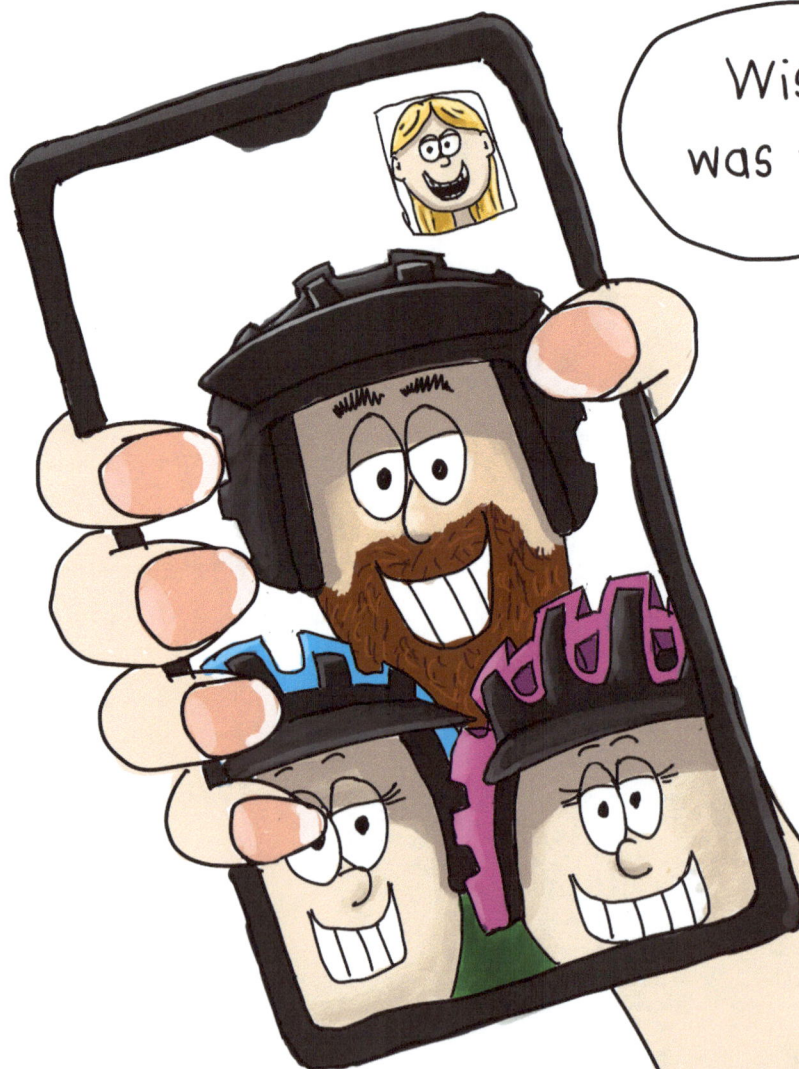

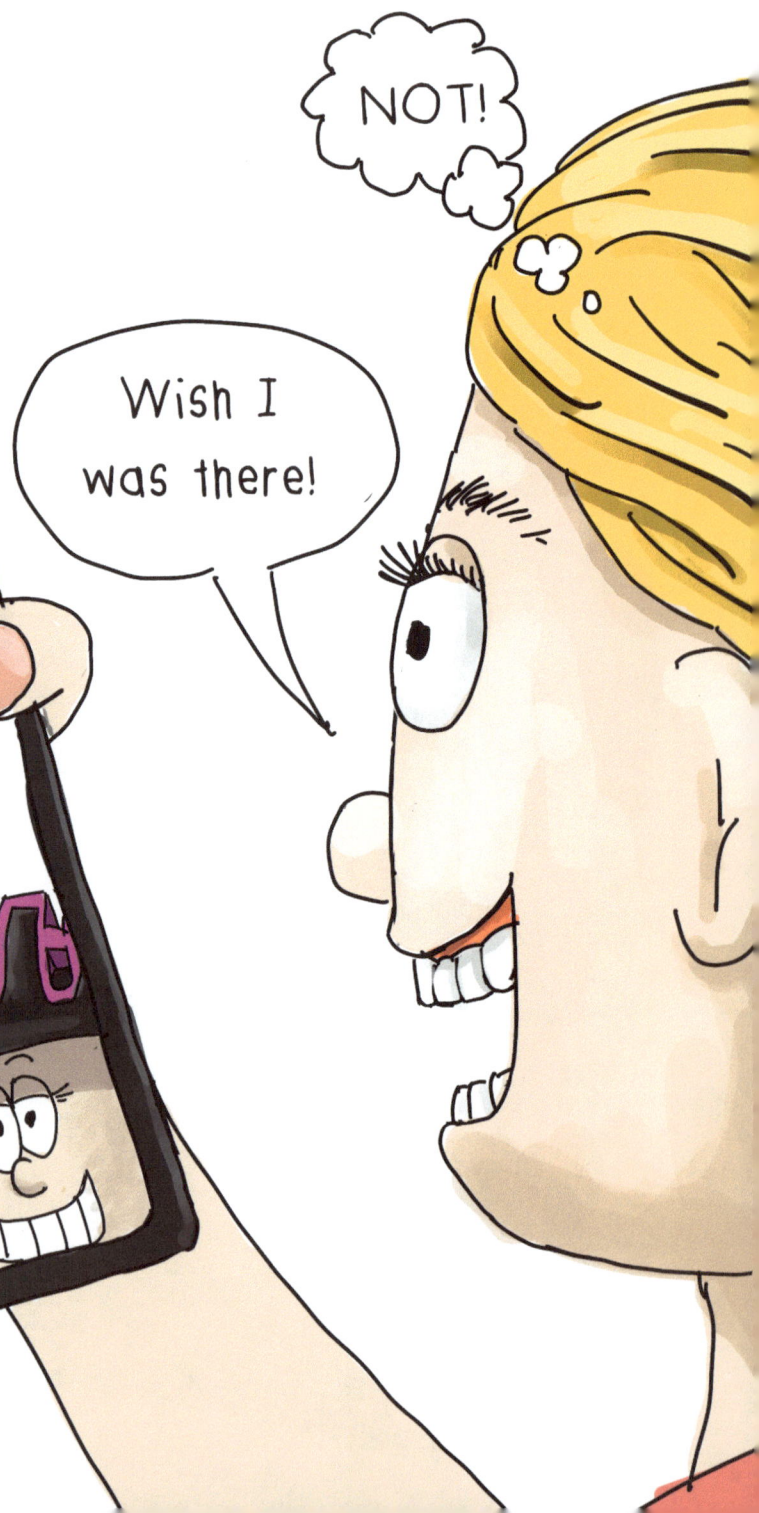

NOT!

Wish I
was there!

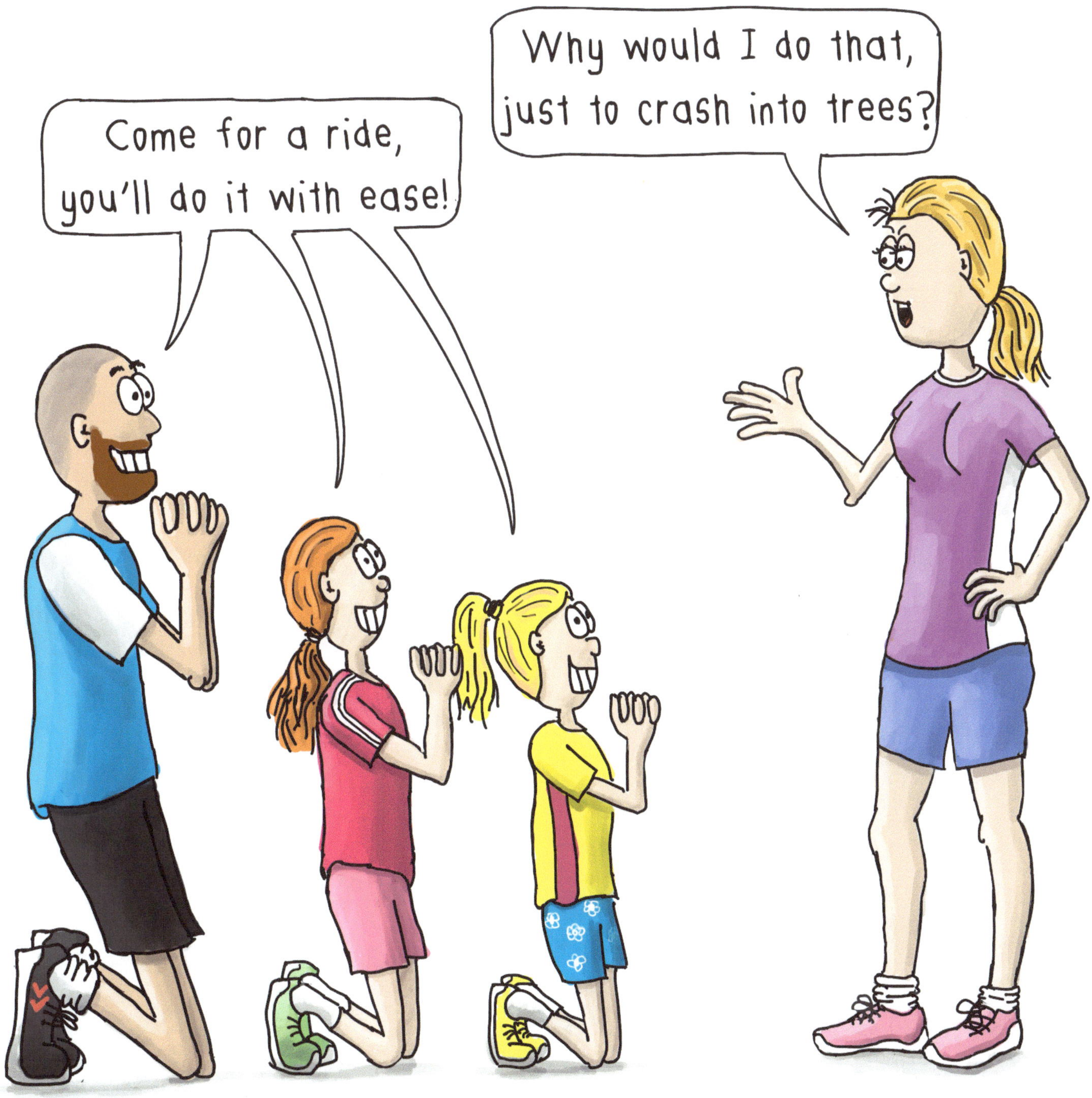
Come for a ride, you'll do it with ease!
Why would I do that, just to crash into trees?

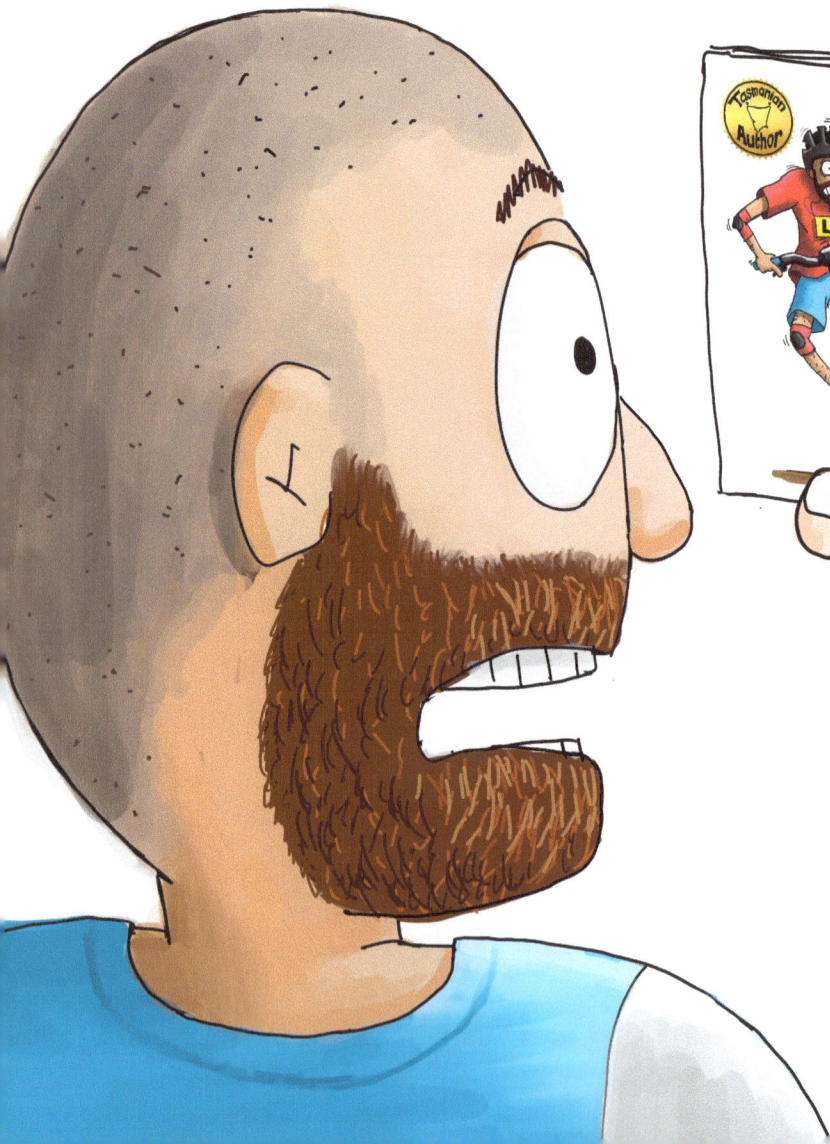

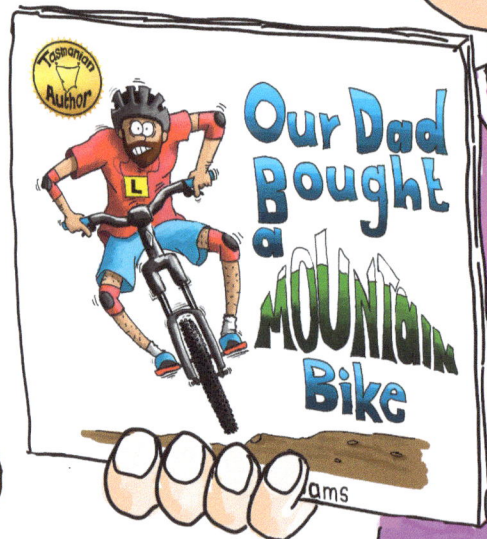

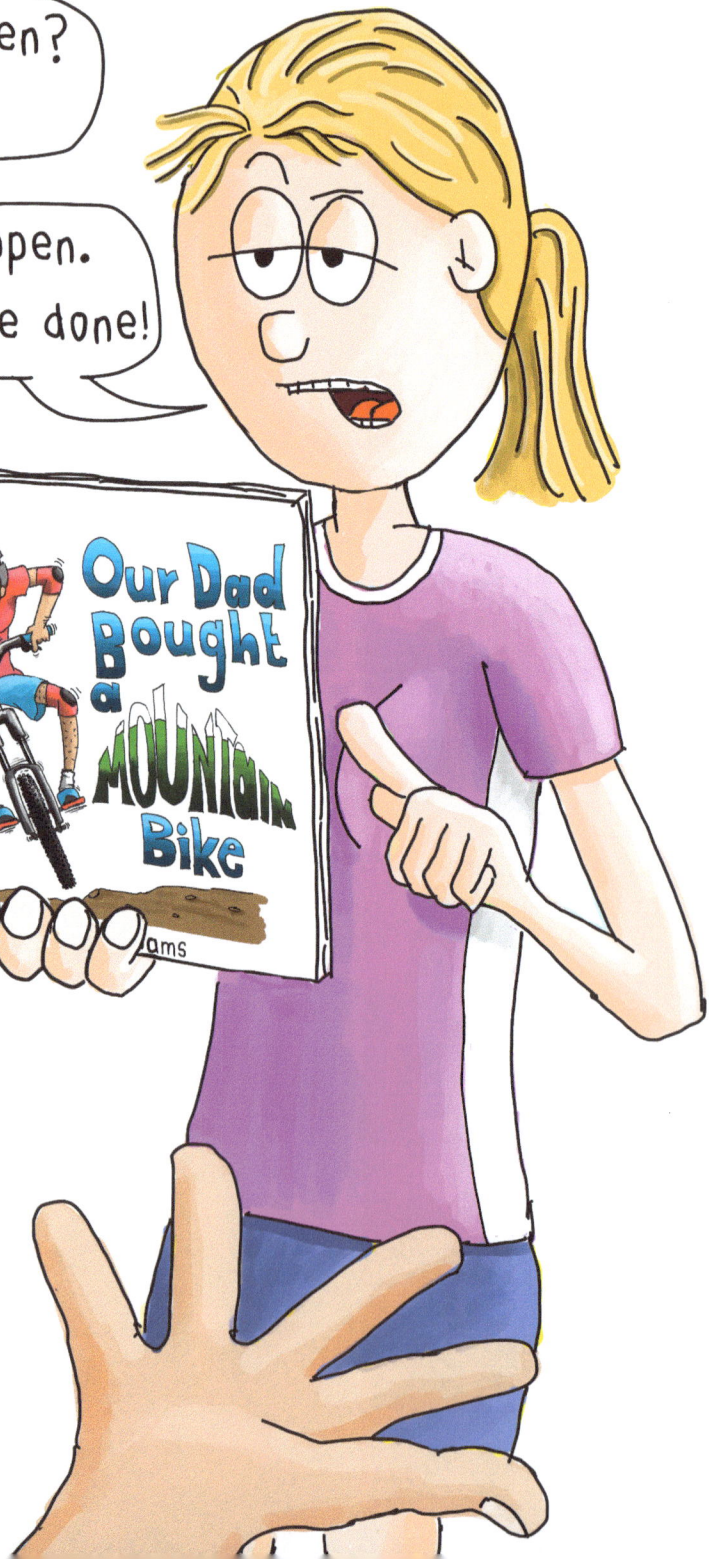

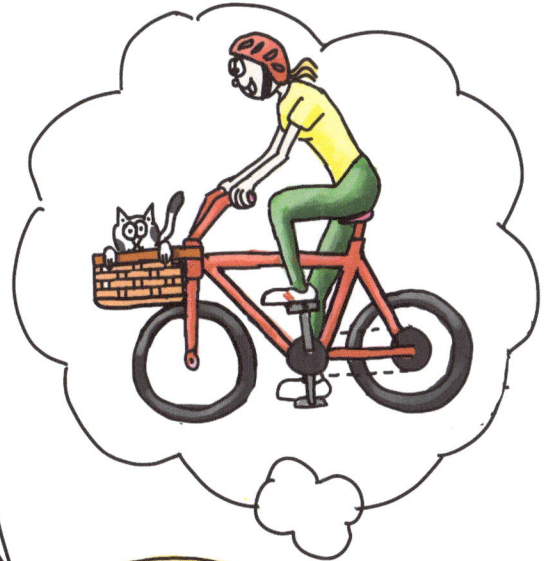

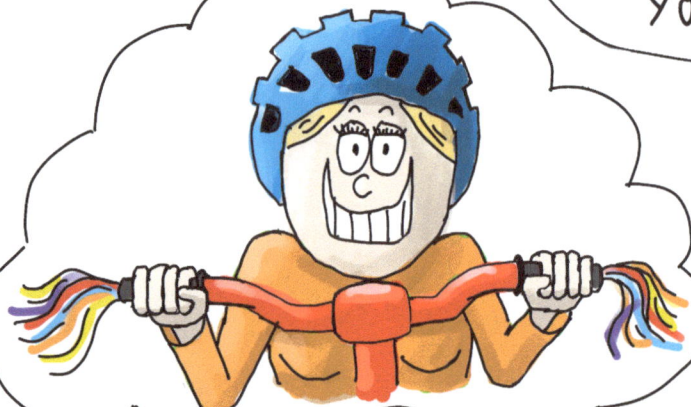

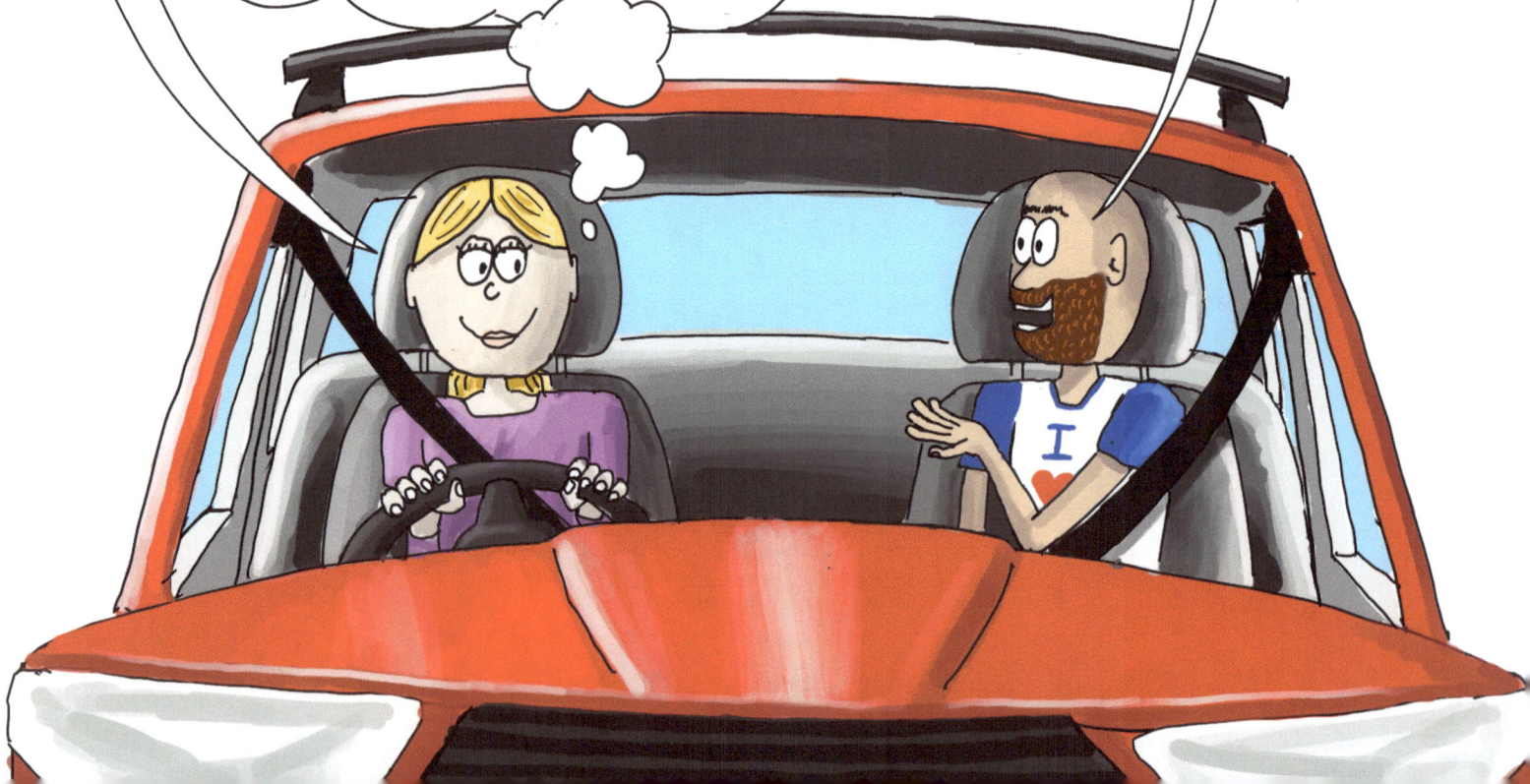

'If I say yes, will it stop you from talking?'
'Groovy,' said Dad, already walking.

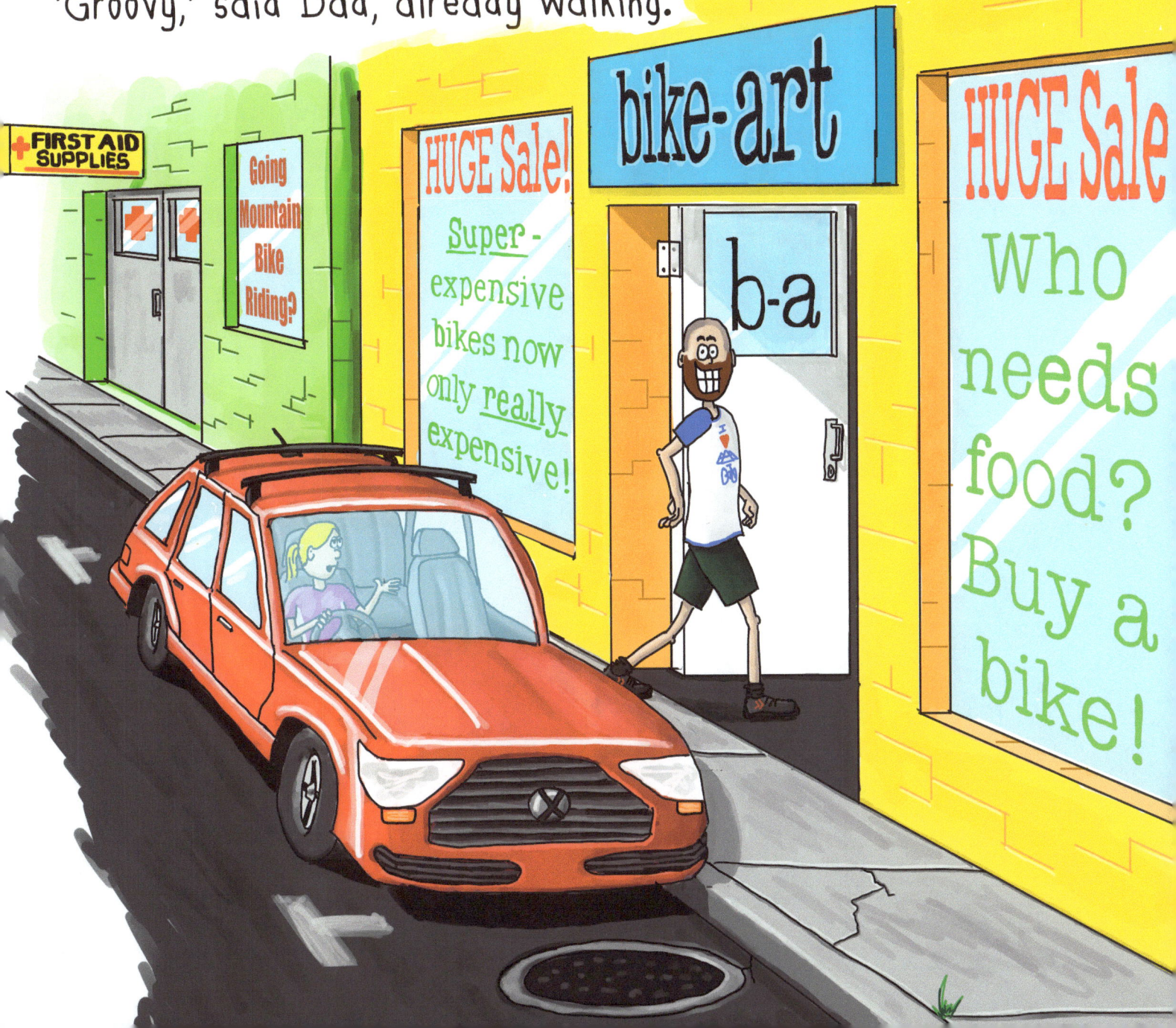

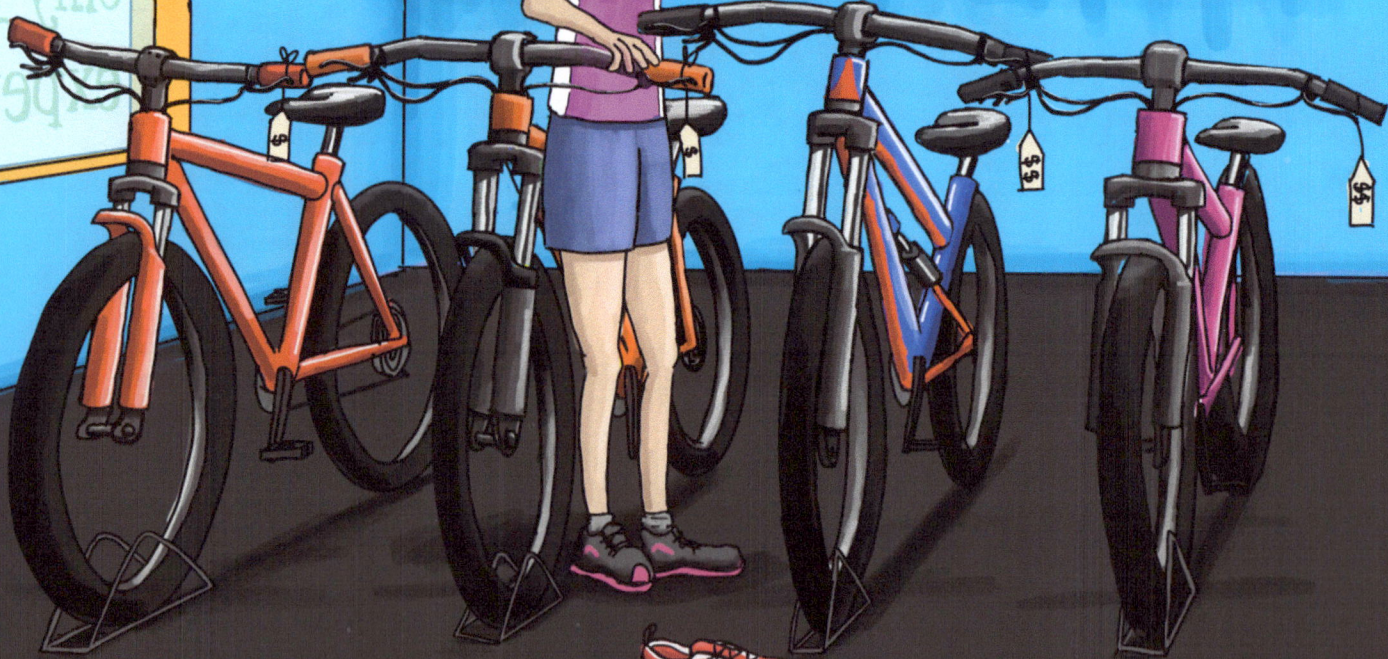

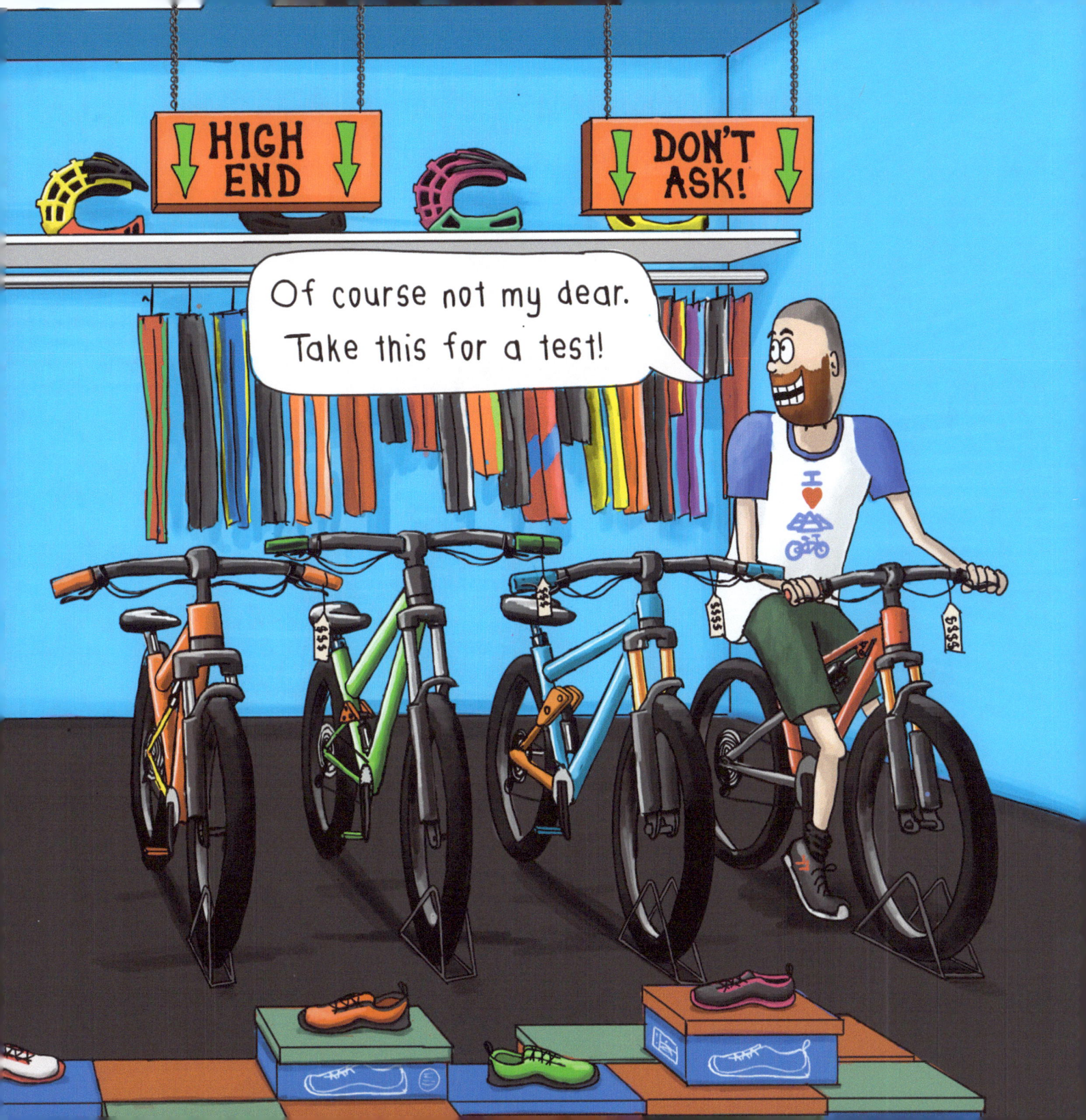

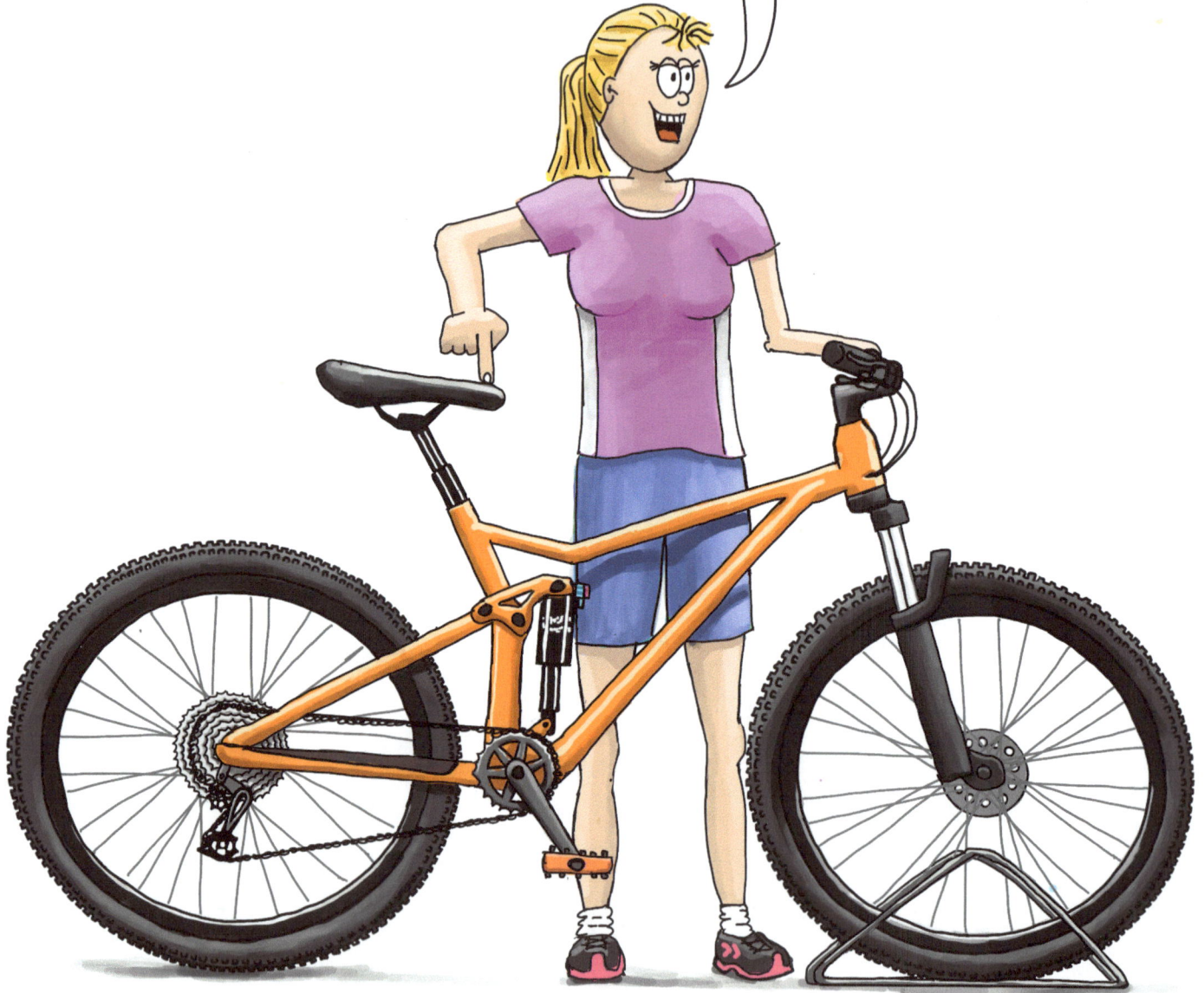

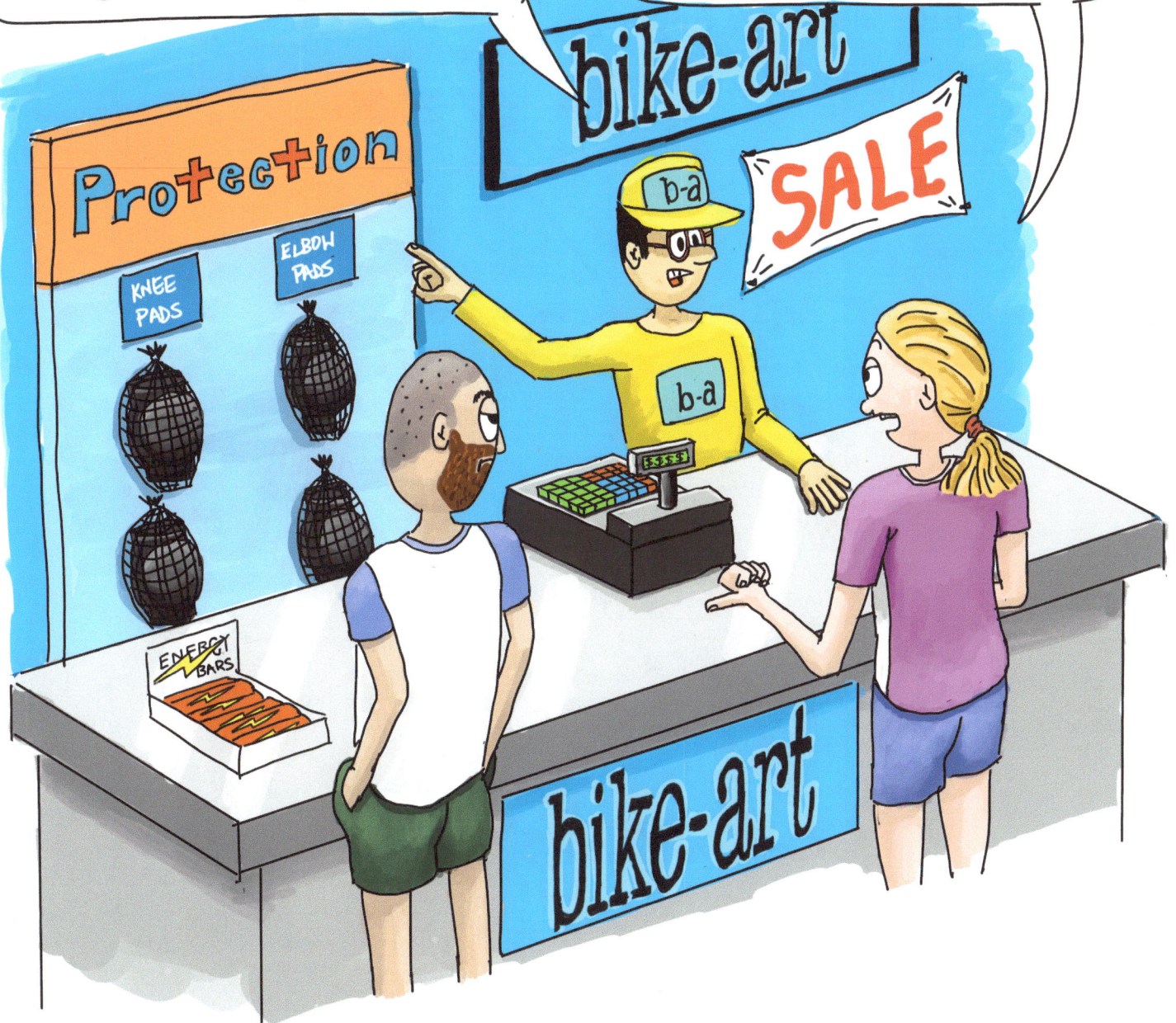

So Mum bought a bike,
not great but not bad.
Unlike Dad, she didn't spend
all the money she had.

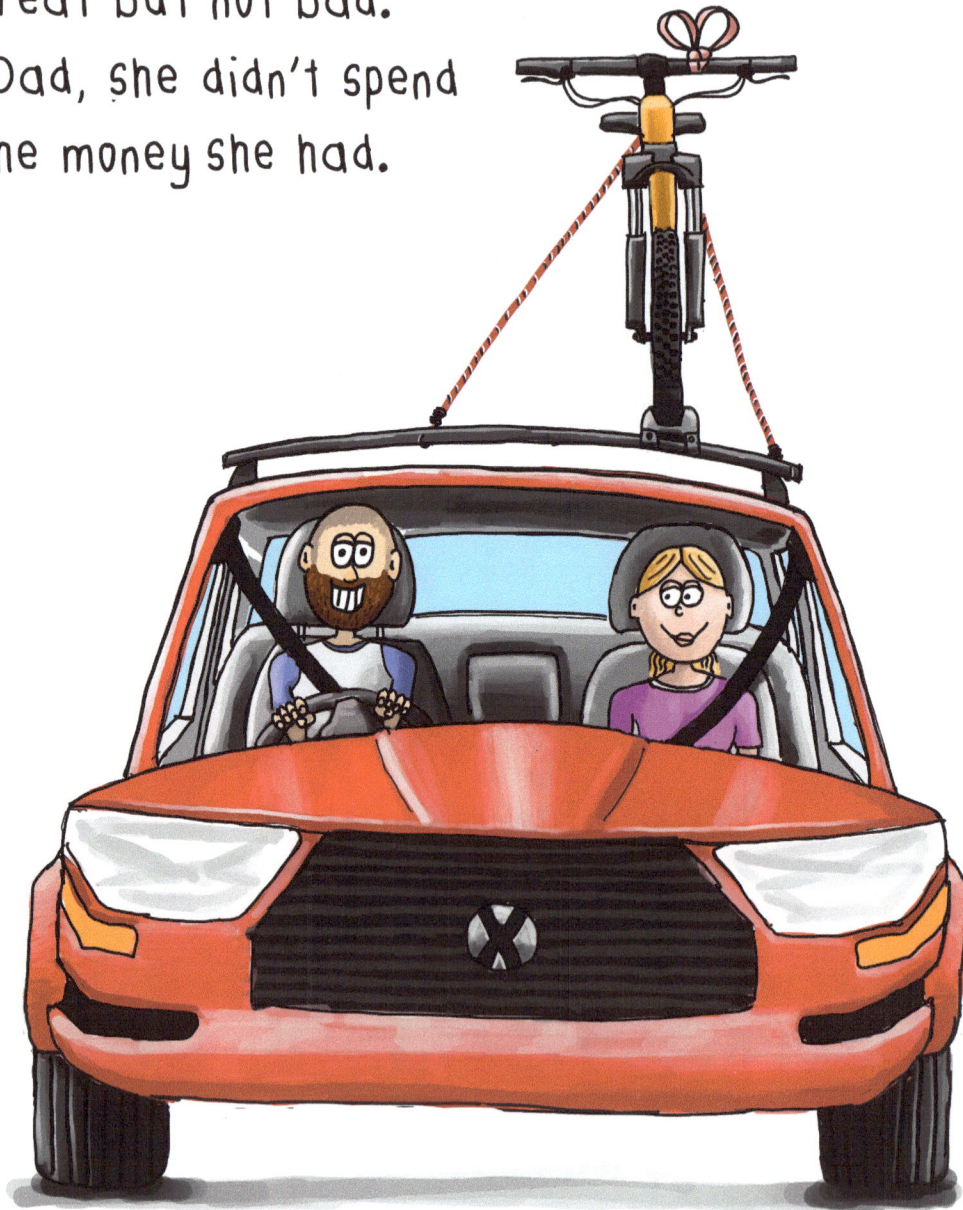

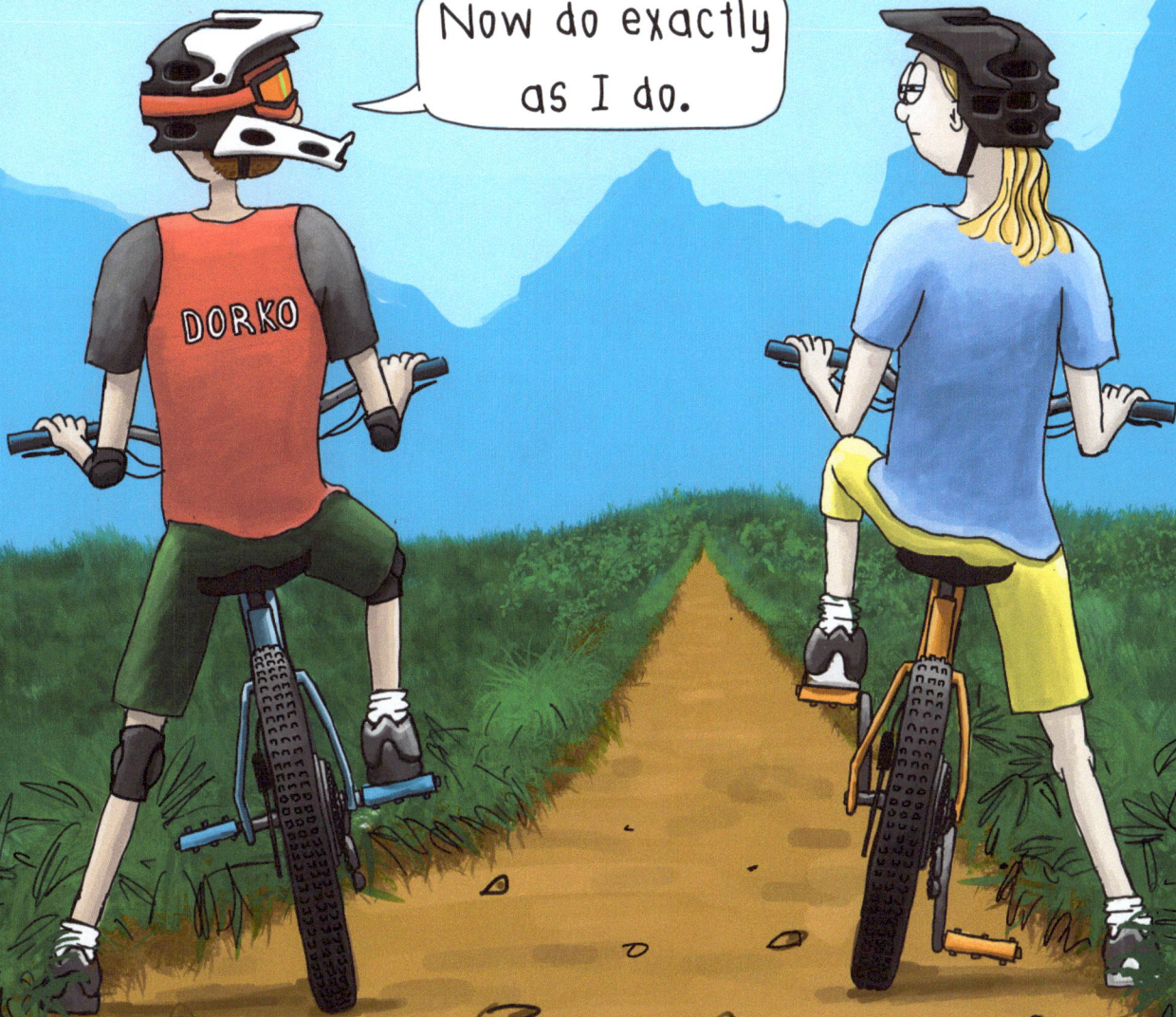

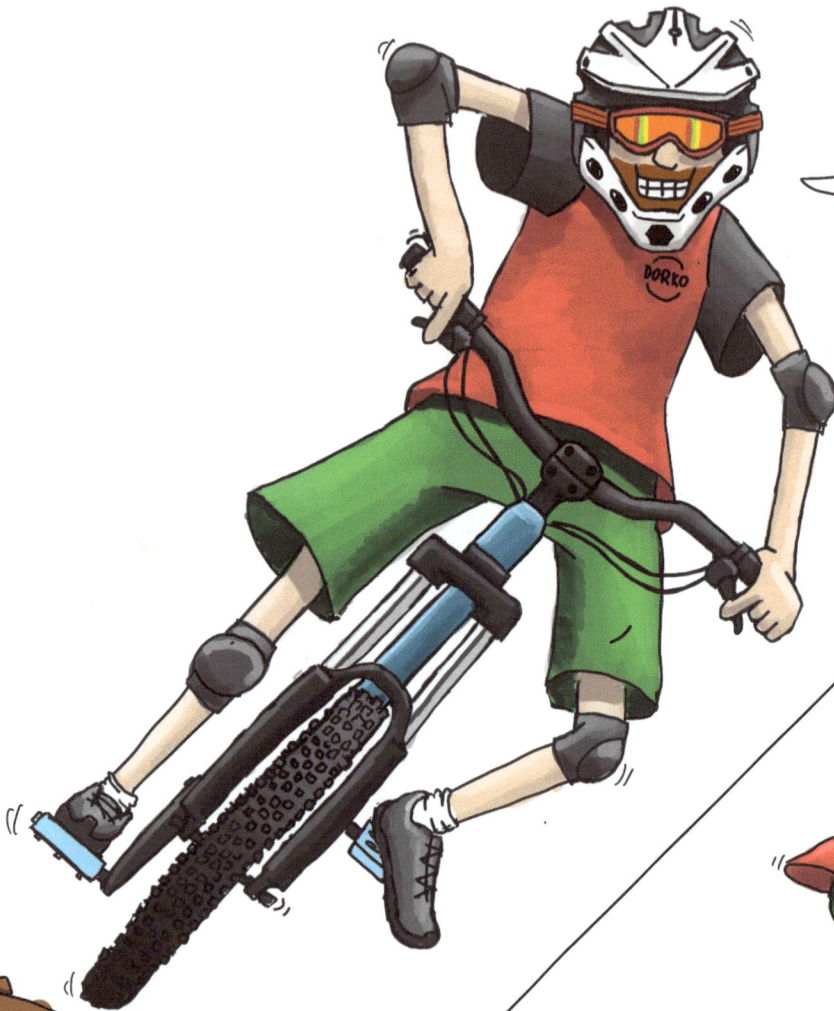

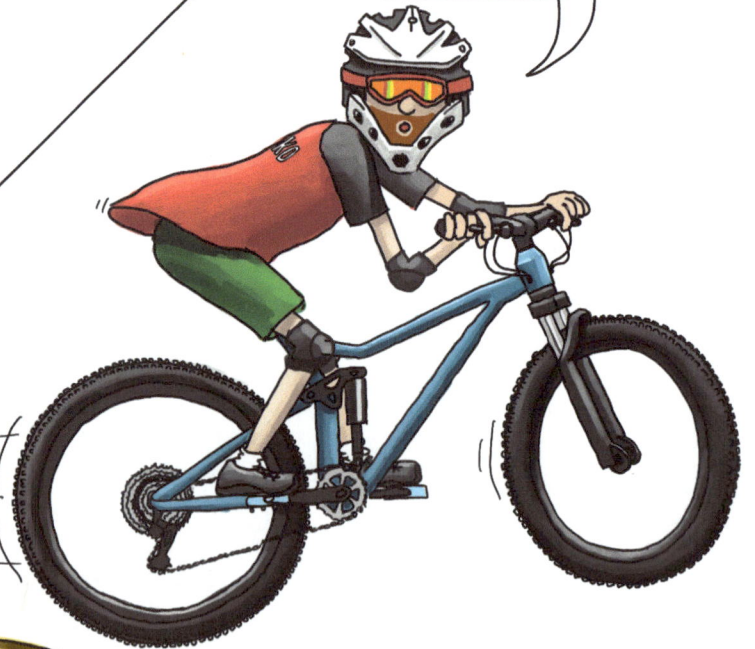

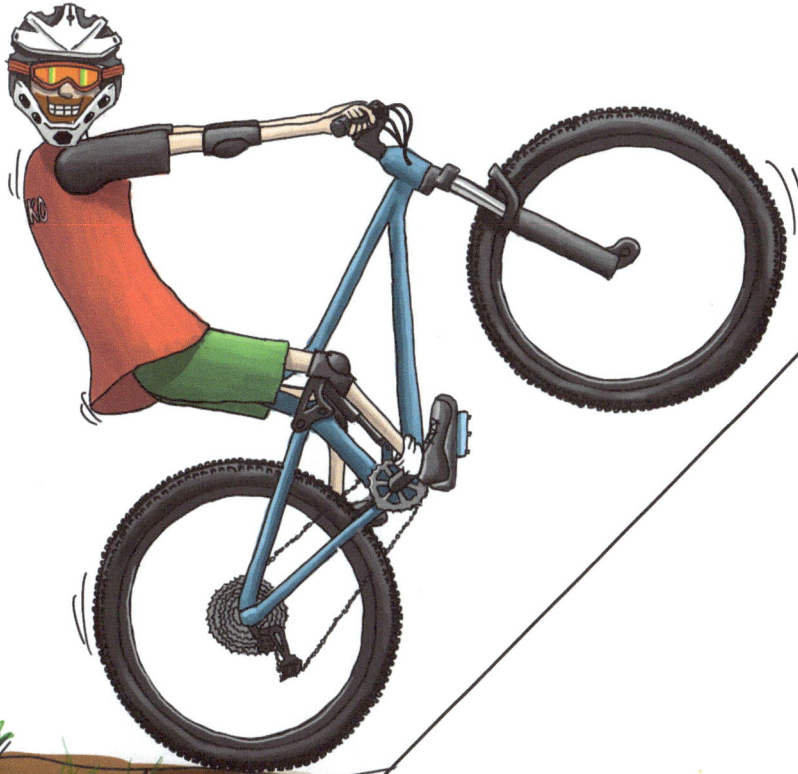

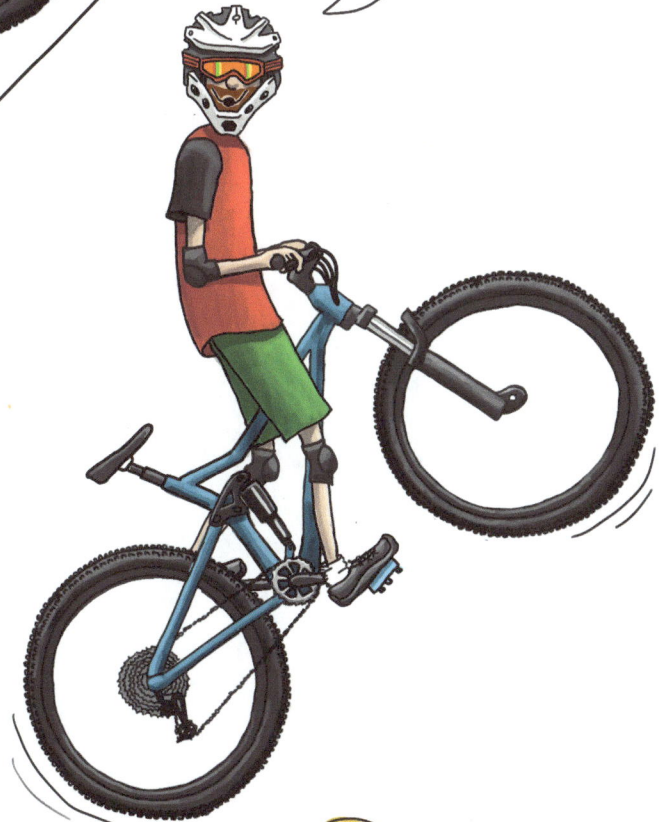

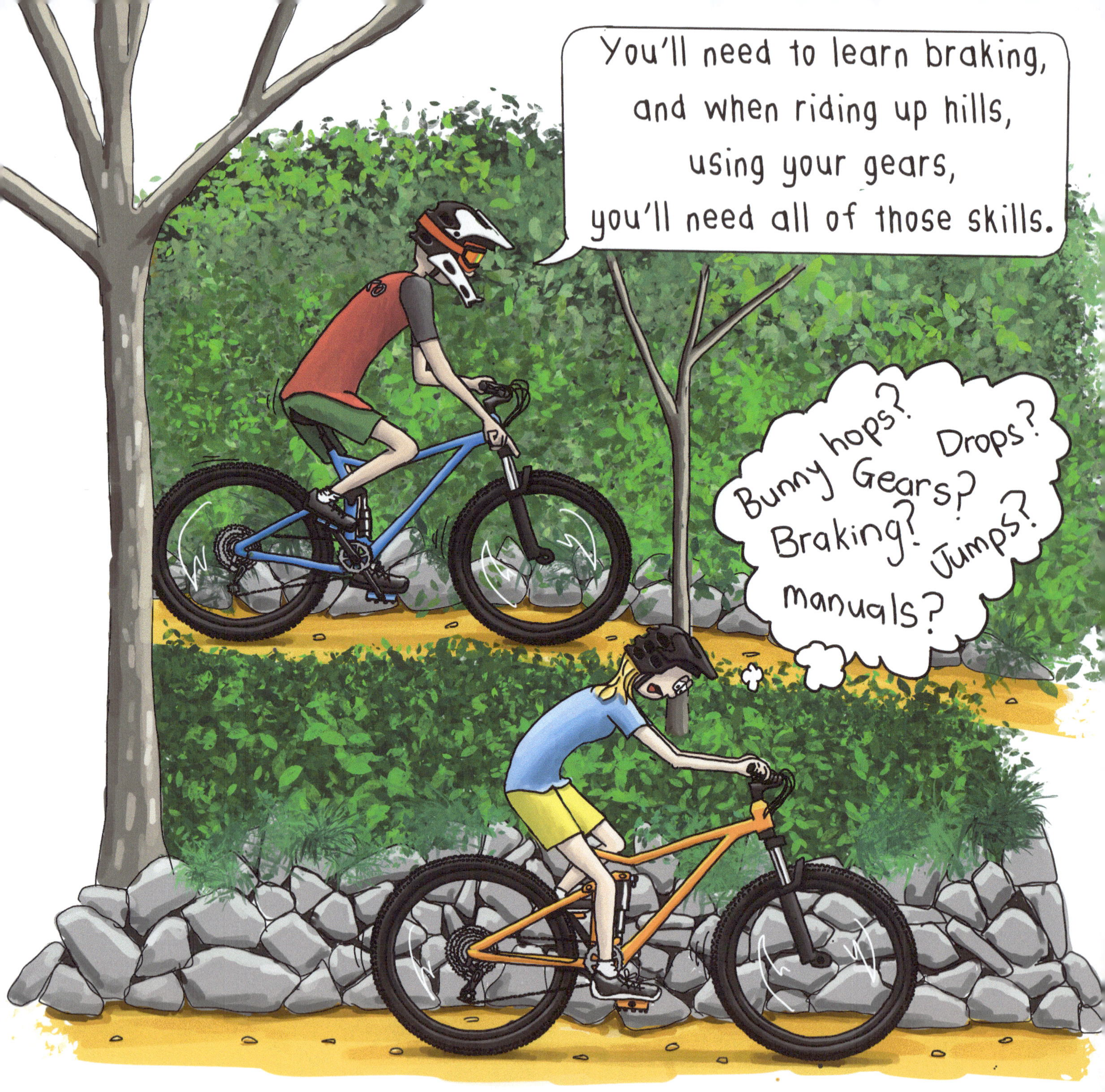
You'll need to learn braking, and when riding up hills, using your gears, you'll need all of those skills.
Bunny hops?
Drops?
Gears?
Braking?
Jumps?
manuals?

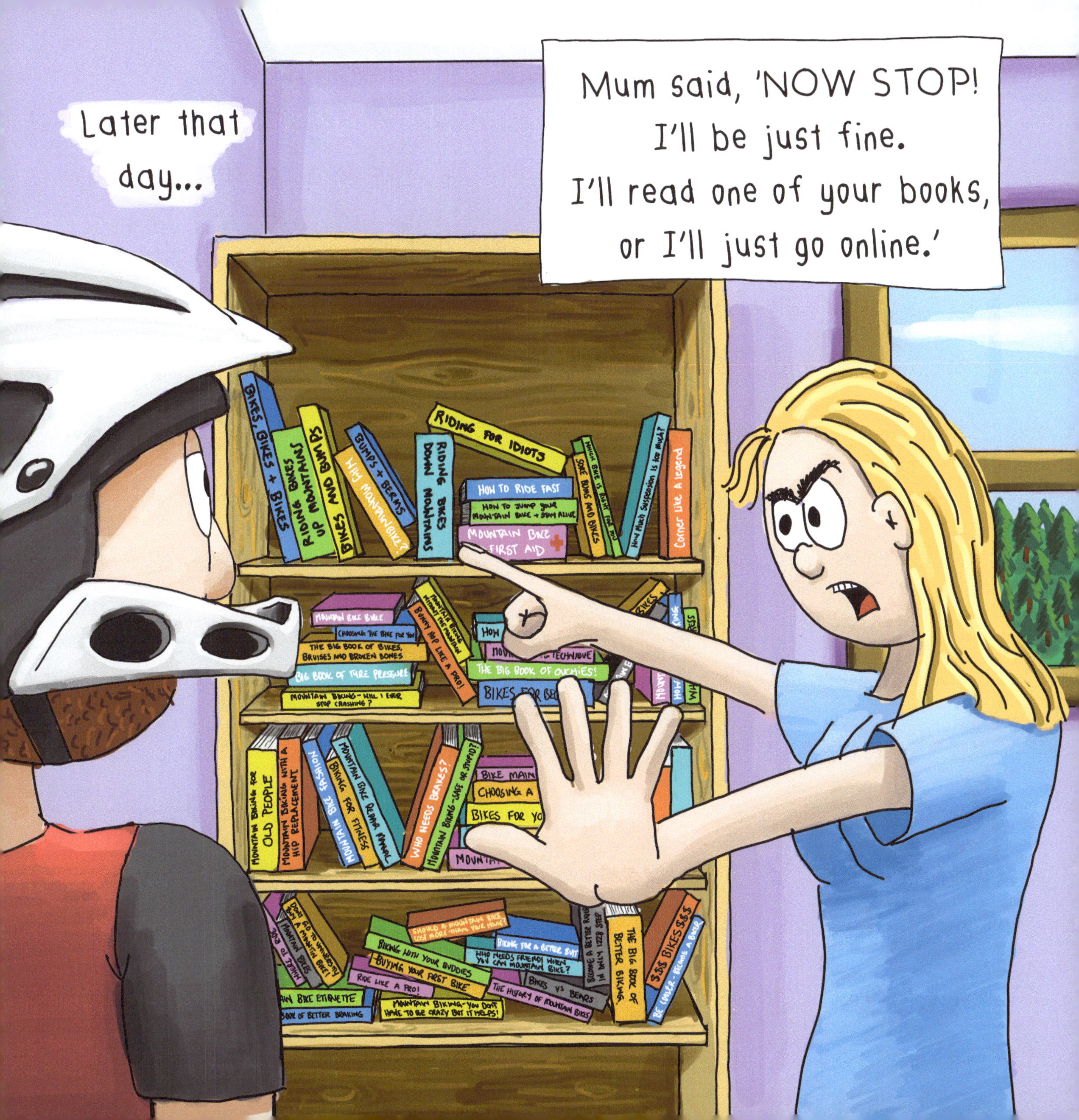
Later that day...
Mum said, 'NOW STOP!
I'll be just fine.
I'll read one of your books,
or I'll just go online.'
BIKES, BIKES + BIKES
RIDING BIKES UP MOUNTAINS
BIKES AND BUMPS
WHY MOUNTAIN BIKE?
BUMPS + BERMS
RIDING BIKES DOWN MOUNTAINS
RIDING FOR IDIOTS
HOW TO RIDE FAST
HOW TO JUMP YOUR MOUNTAIN BIKE + STAY ALIVE
MOUNTAIN BIKE FIRST AID
SORE BUMS AND BIKES
How Much Suspension is too Much?
Corner Like A Legend
MOUNTAIN BIKE BIBLE
CHOOSING THE BIKE FOR YOU
THE BIG BOOK OF BIKES, BRUISES AND BROKEN BONES
BIG BOOK OF TYRE PRESSURE
MOUNTAIN BIKING - WILL I EVER STOP CRASHING?
BUNNY HOP LIKE A PRO!
THE BIG BOOK OF OUCHIES!
MOUNTAIN BIKING FOR OLD PEOPLE
MOUNTAIN BIKING WITH A HIP REPLACEMENT
MOUNTAIN BIKE FASHION
BIKING FOR FITNESS
MOUNTAIN BIKE REPAIR MANUAL
WHO NEEDS BRAKES?
MOUNTAIN BIKING - SAFE OR STUPID?
SHOULD A MOUNTAIN BIKE COST MORE THAN YOUR HOME?
BIKING FOR A BETTER BUTT
WHO NEEDS FRIENDS WHEN YOU CAN MOUNTAIN BIKE?
BIKING WITH YOUR BUDDIES
BUYING YOUR FIRST BIKE
RIDE LIKE A PRO!
BIKES VS BEARS
THE HISTORY OF MOUNTAIN BIKES
MOUNTAIN BIKING - YOU DON'T HAVE TO BE CRAZY BUT IT HELPS!
THE BIG BOOK OF BETTER BIKING
$$$ BIKES $$$
BE COOLER - BECOME A BIKER

So Mum took her bike
to ride off to the track.
She'd just left the house,
when she had her first stack.

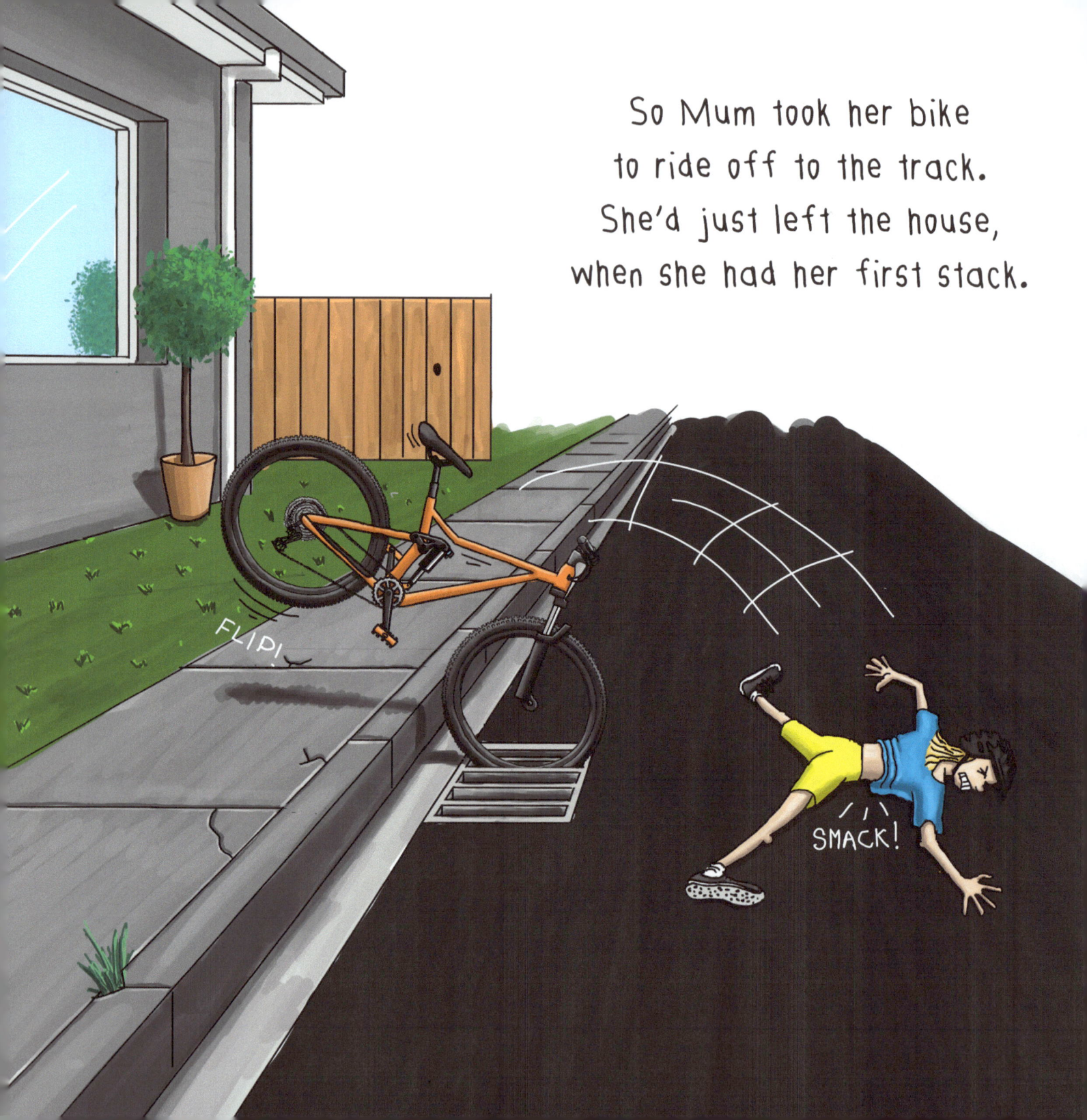

FLIP!

SMACK!

And so it went on,
Mum would ride every day.
At night she'd read books,
but she'd crash anyway!

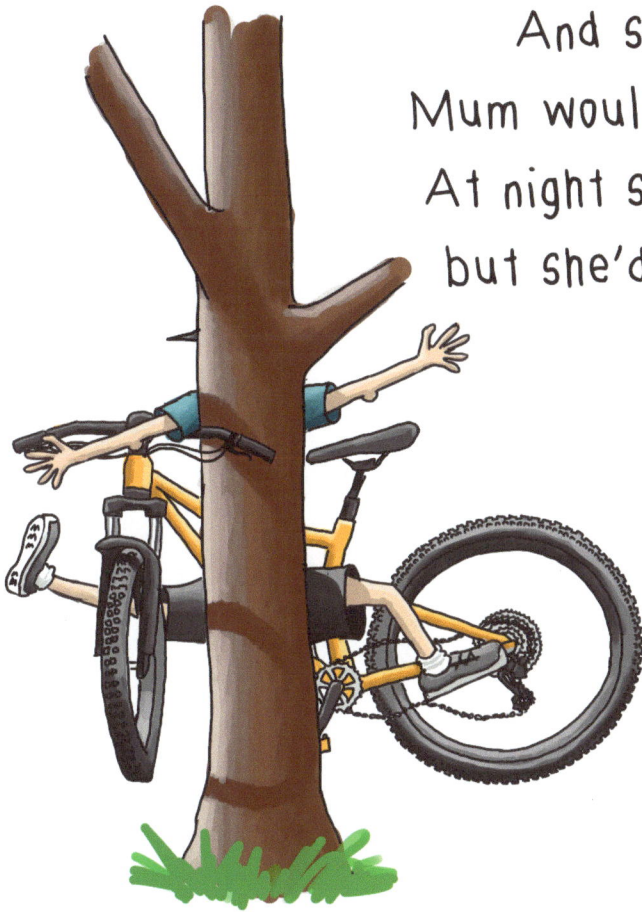

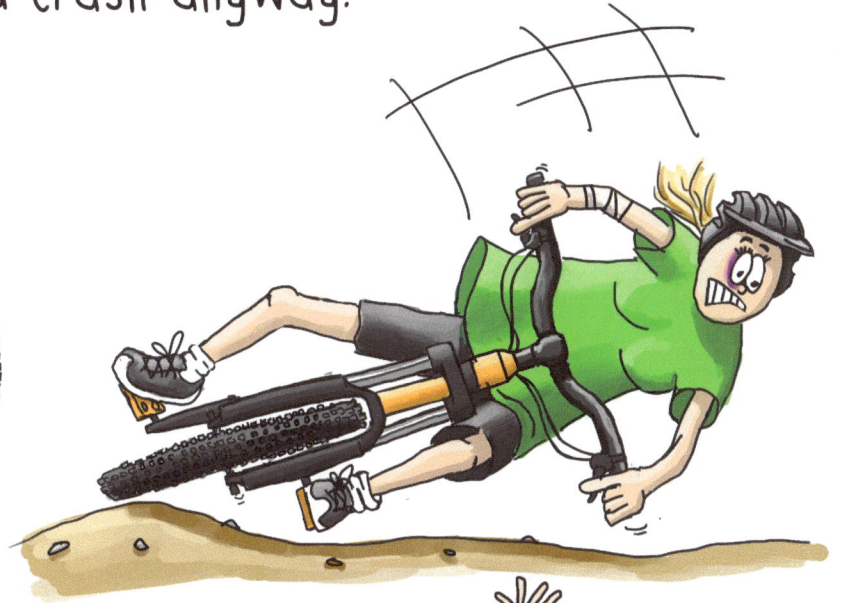

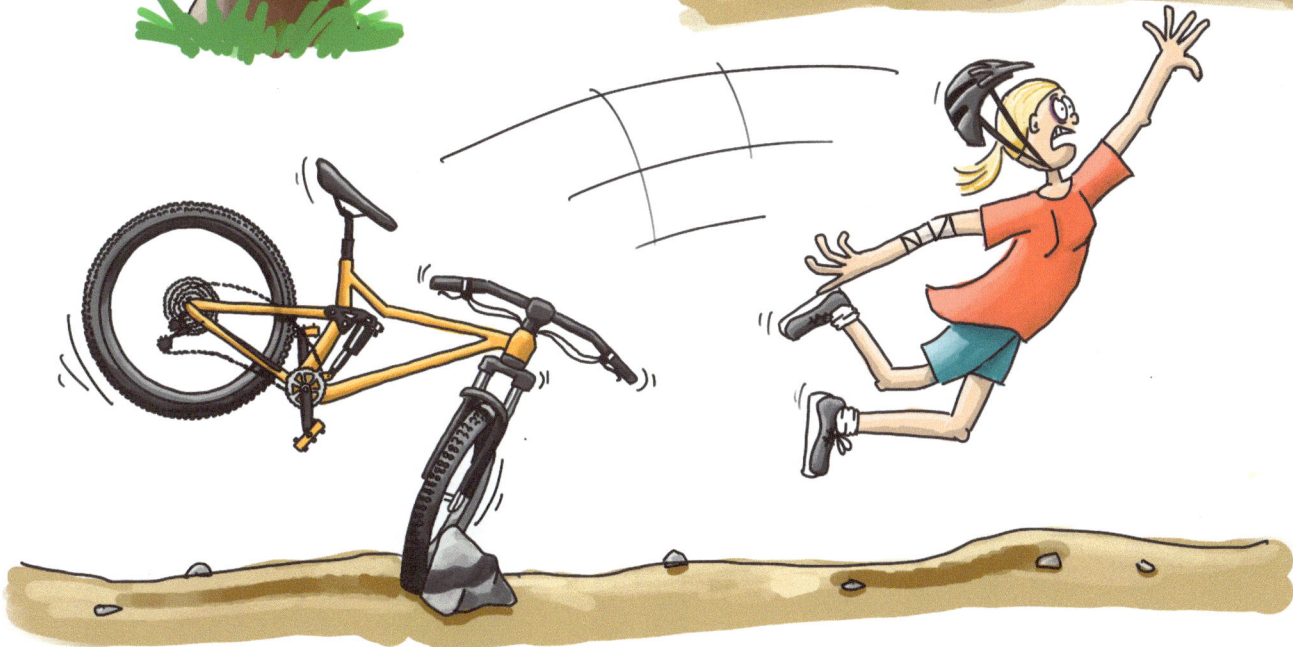

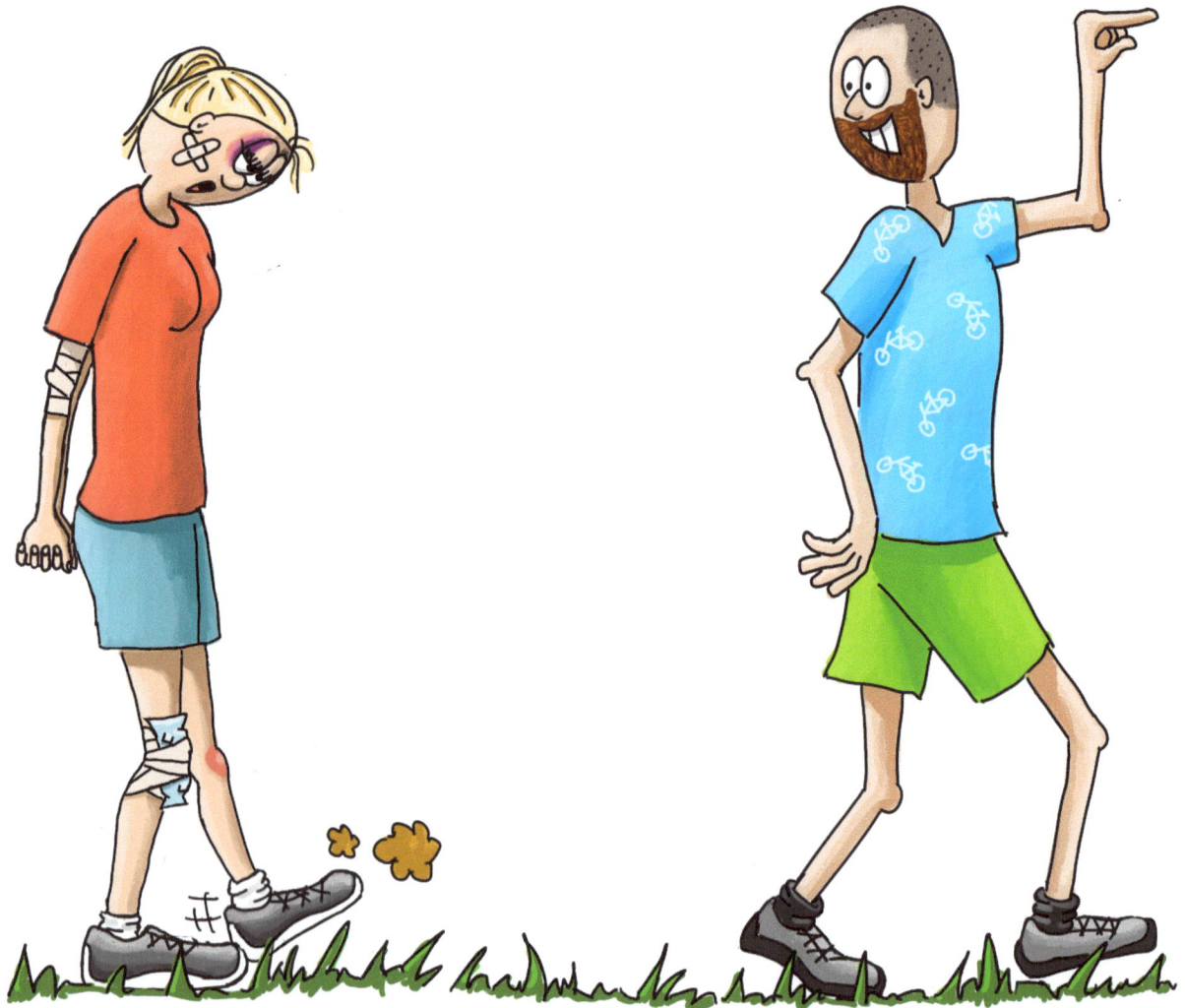

So Dad taught Mum cornering,
and riding up hills,
and bunny hops, and manuals.
She learned all of those skills.

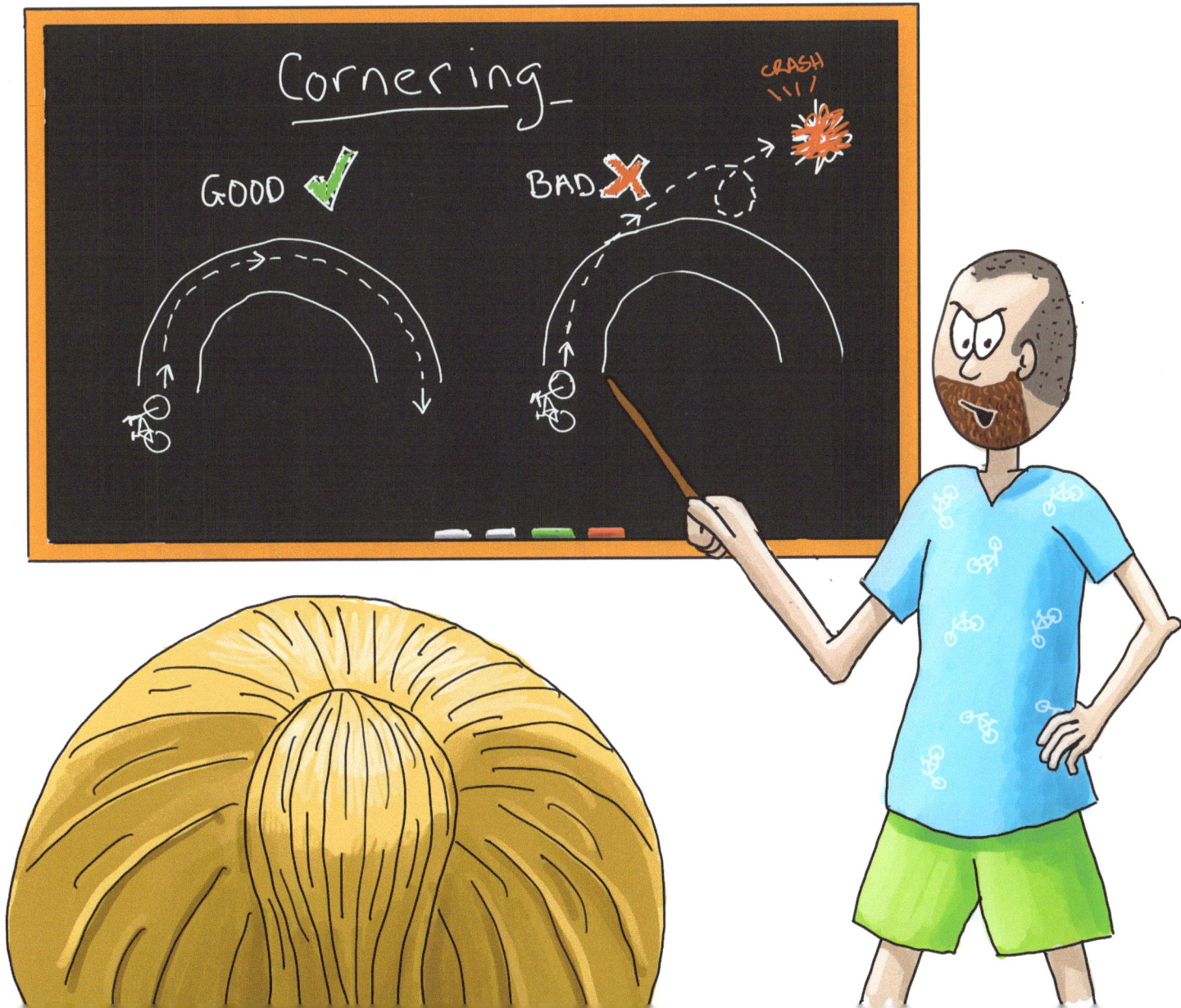

Dad then taught her drops,
and how to do jumps.
And moving her body
to ride fast over bumps.

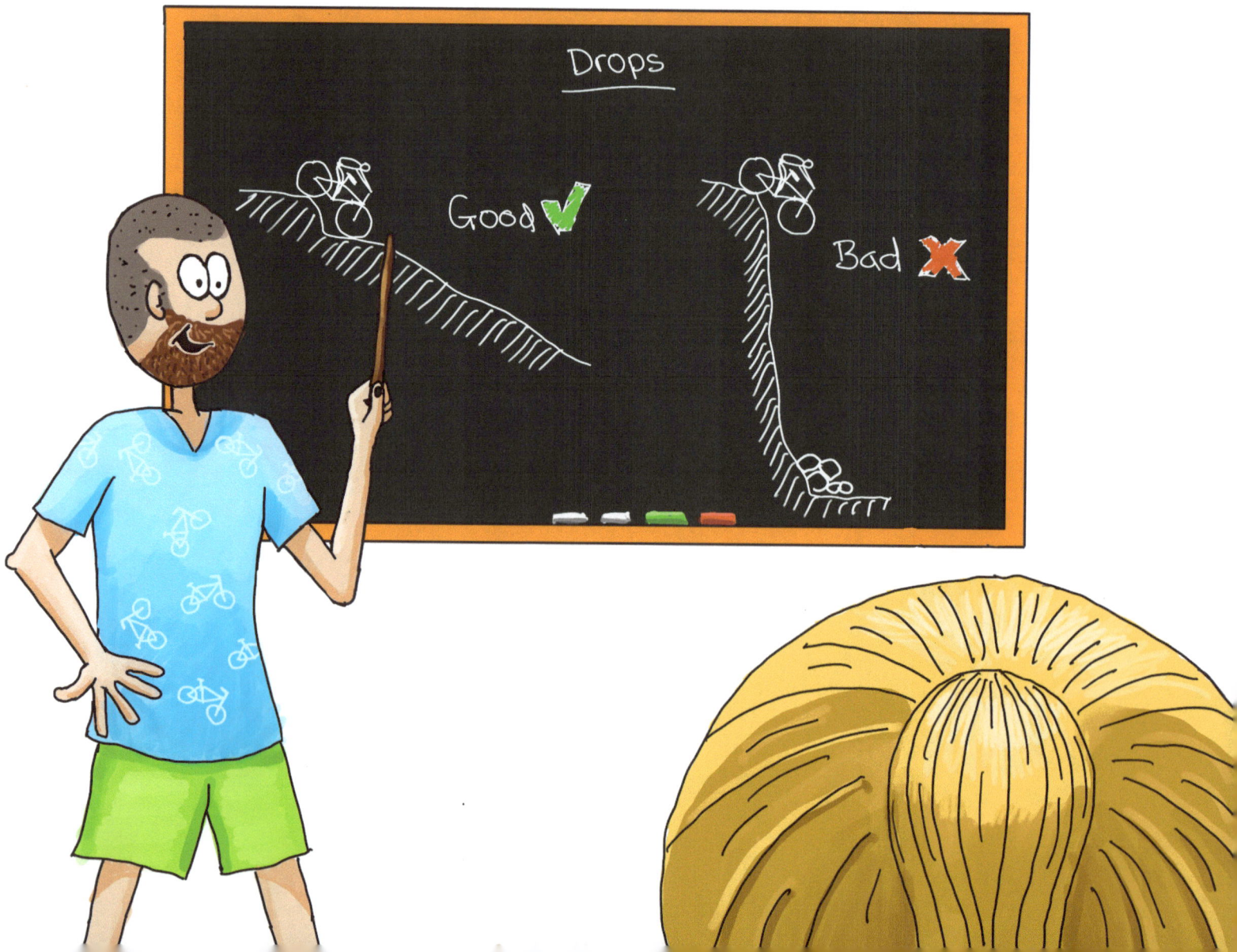

Mum even got pads
for her elbows and knees,
in case she became
too familiar with trees.

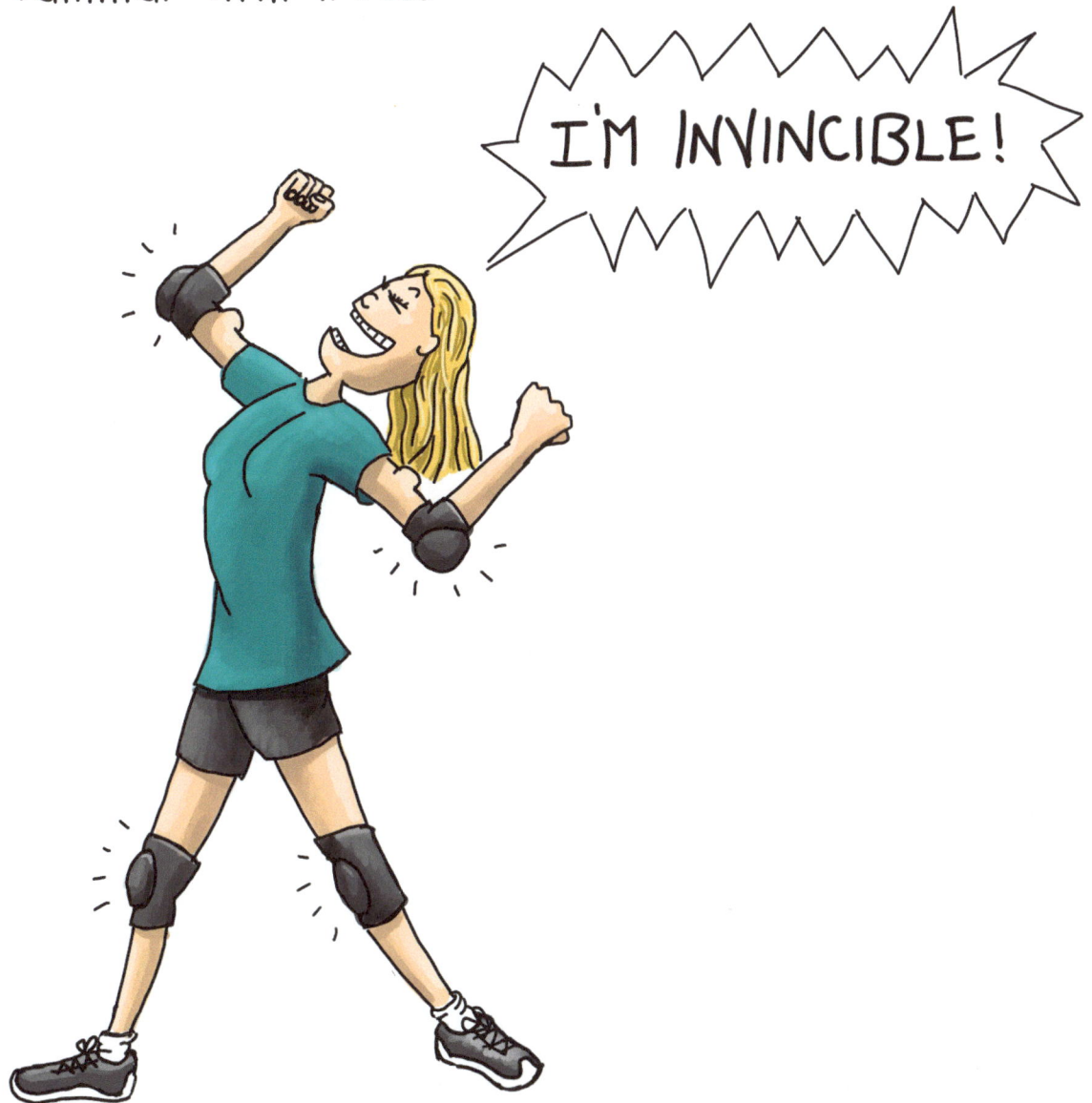

So Mum took the skills, she learnt from our dad,
up into the mountains and she wasn't too bad!

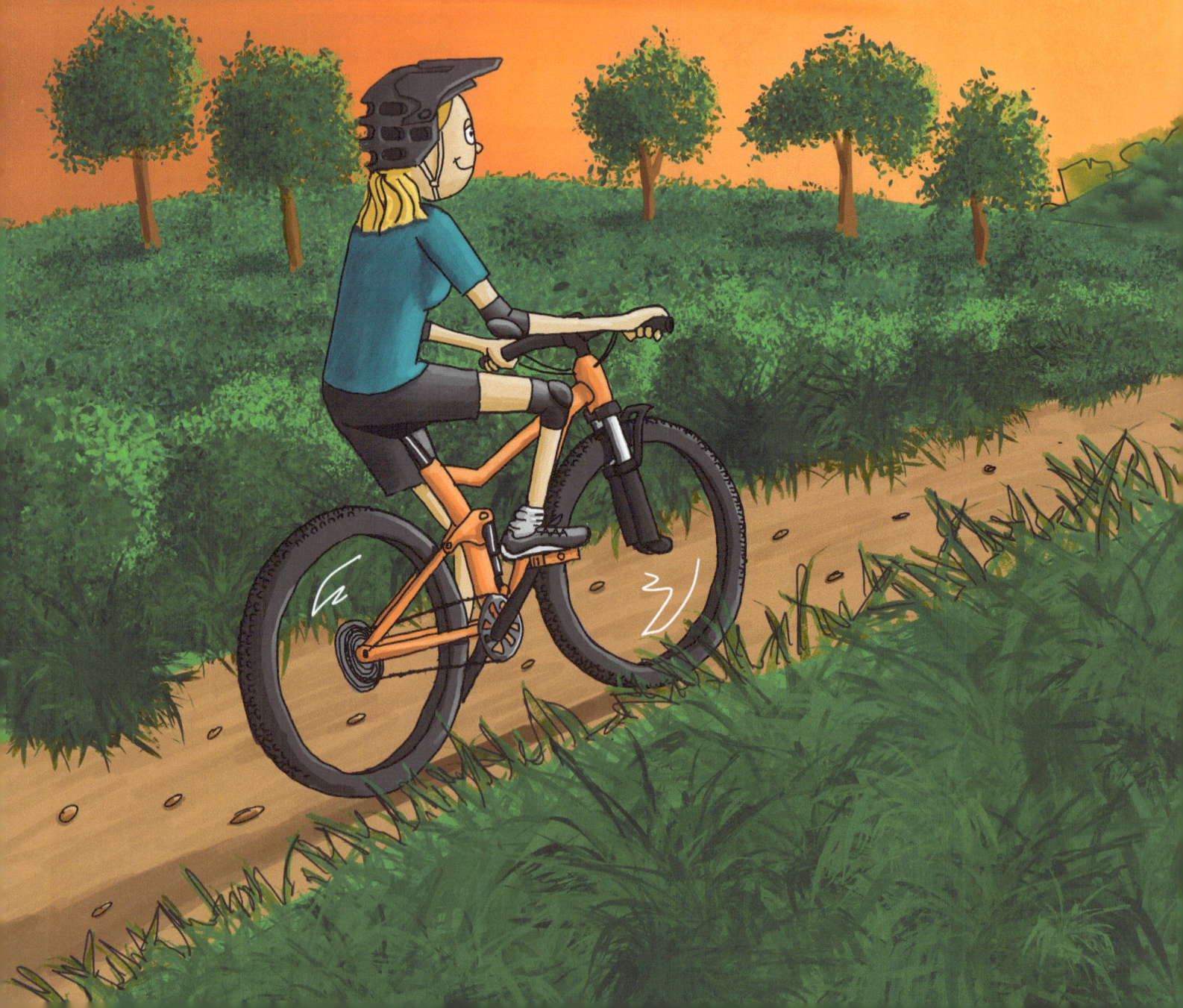

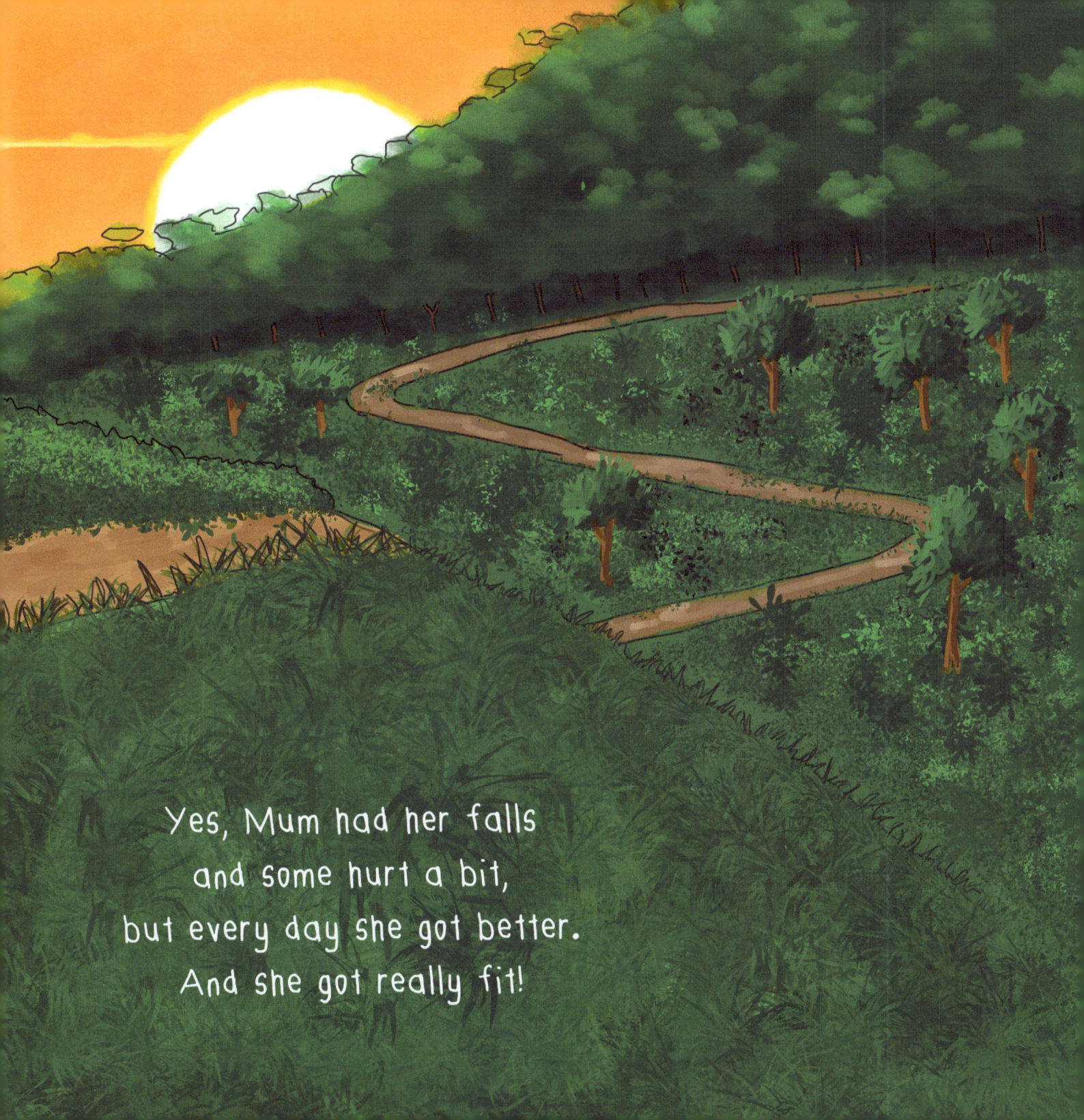

Yes, Mum had her falls
and some hurt a bit,
but every day she got better.
And she got really fit!

START START START START START START START ST

Before too long,
Mum had entered a race.
Dad said, 'Be careful,
don't try for my pace.'

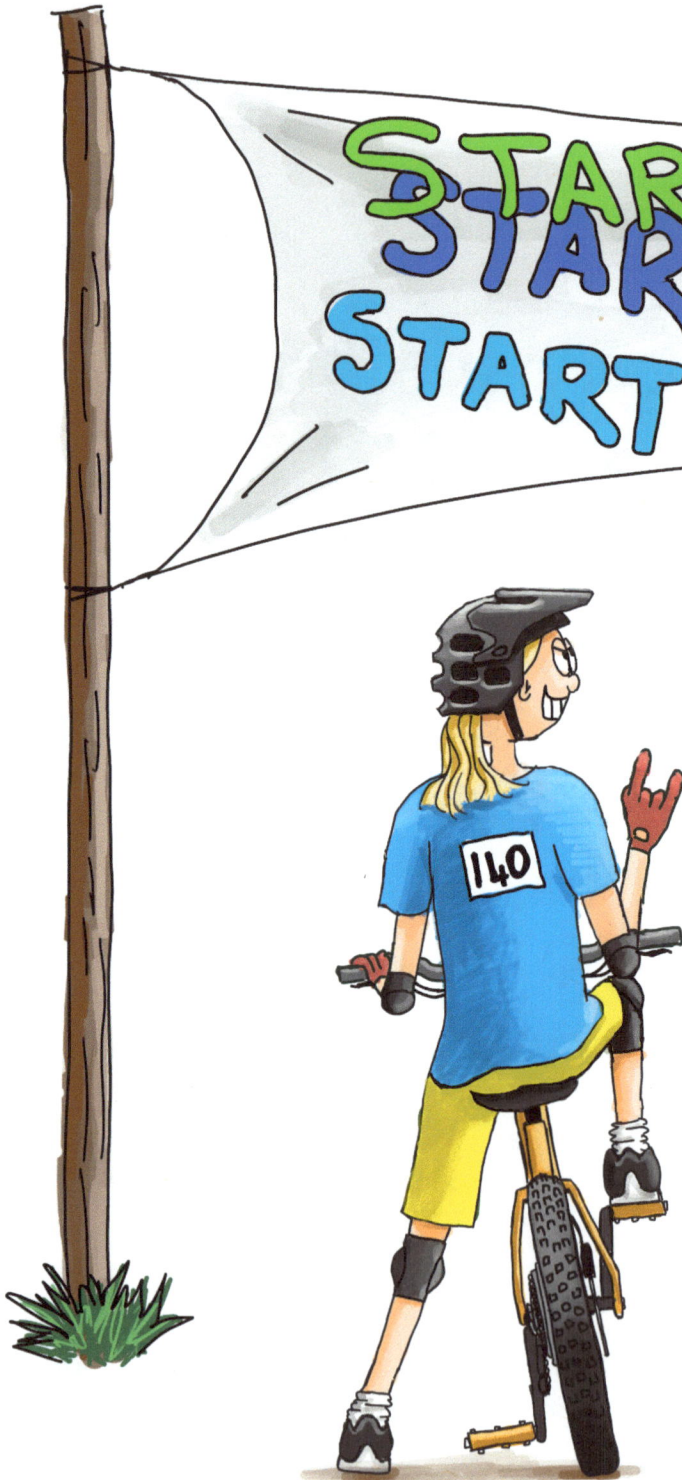

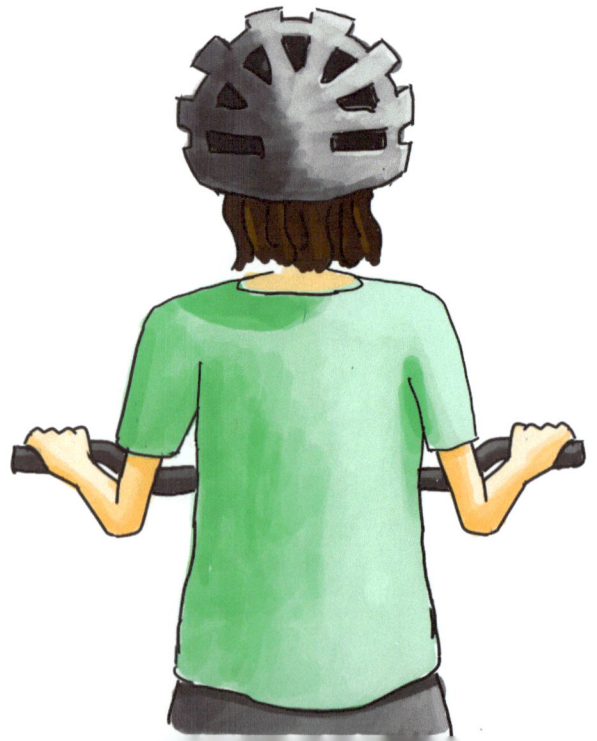

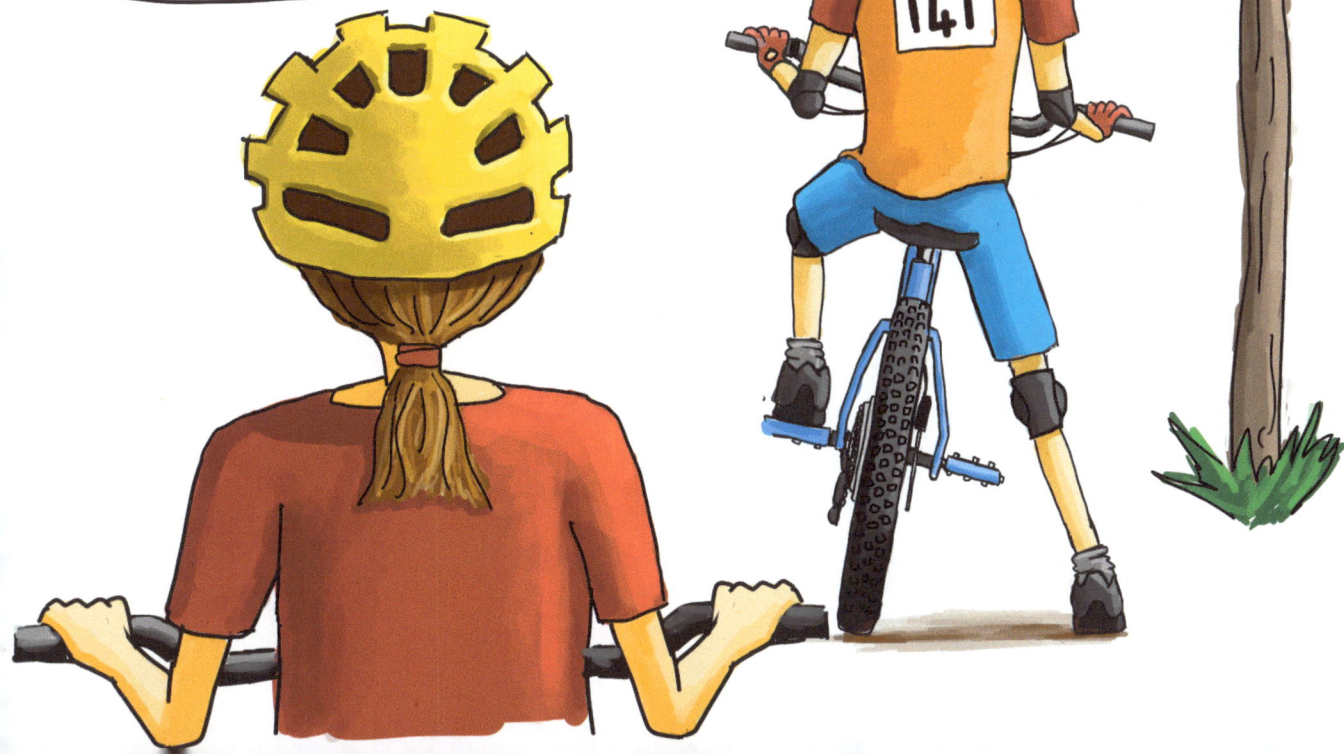

But Mum had worked hard,
and knew just how to send.
No way she'd let Dad
beat her to the end.

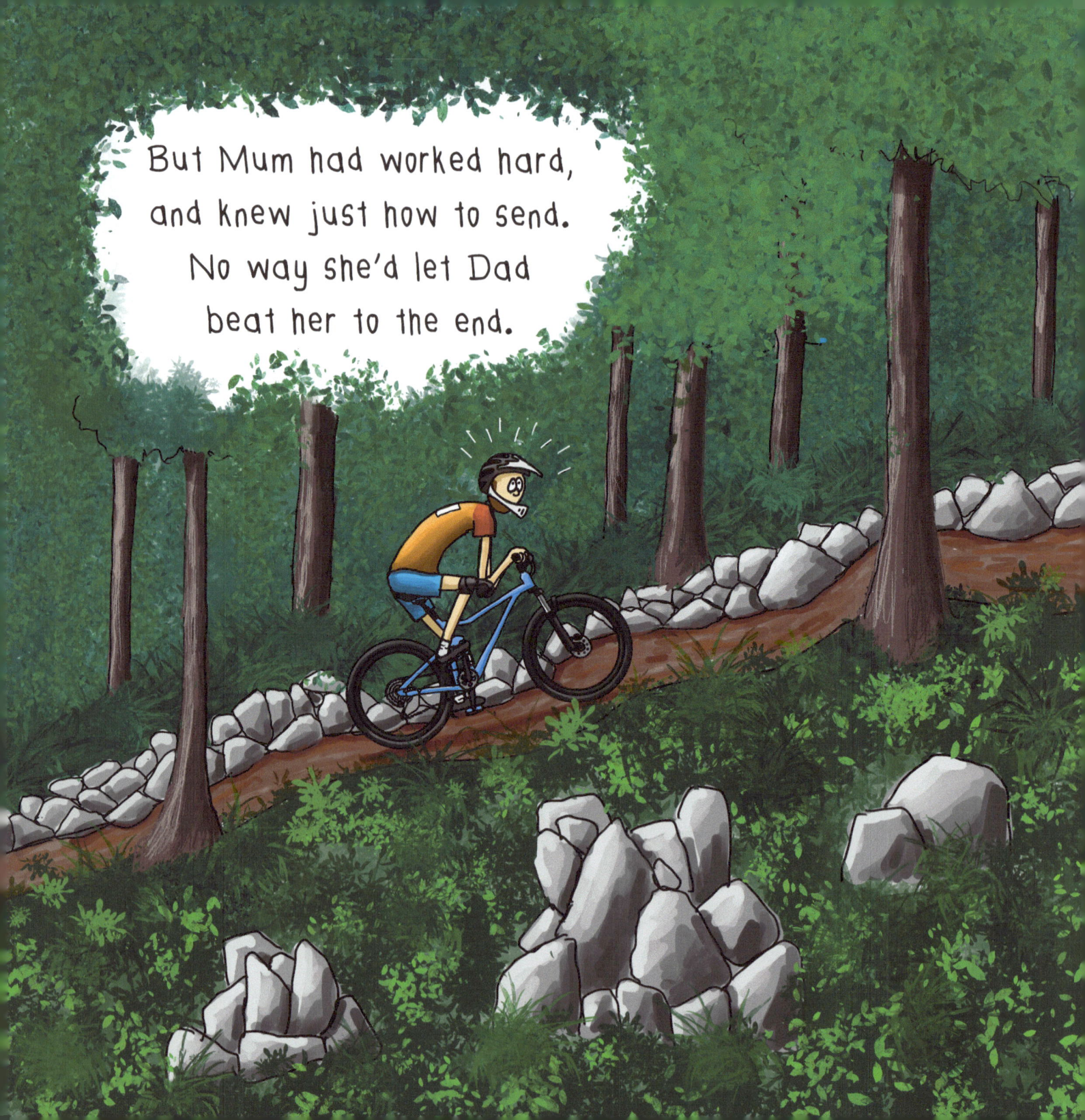

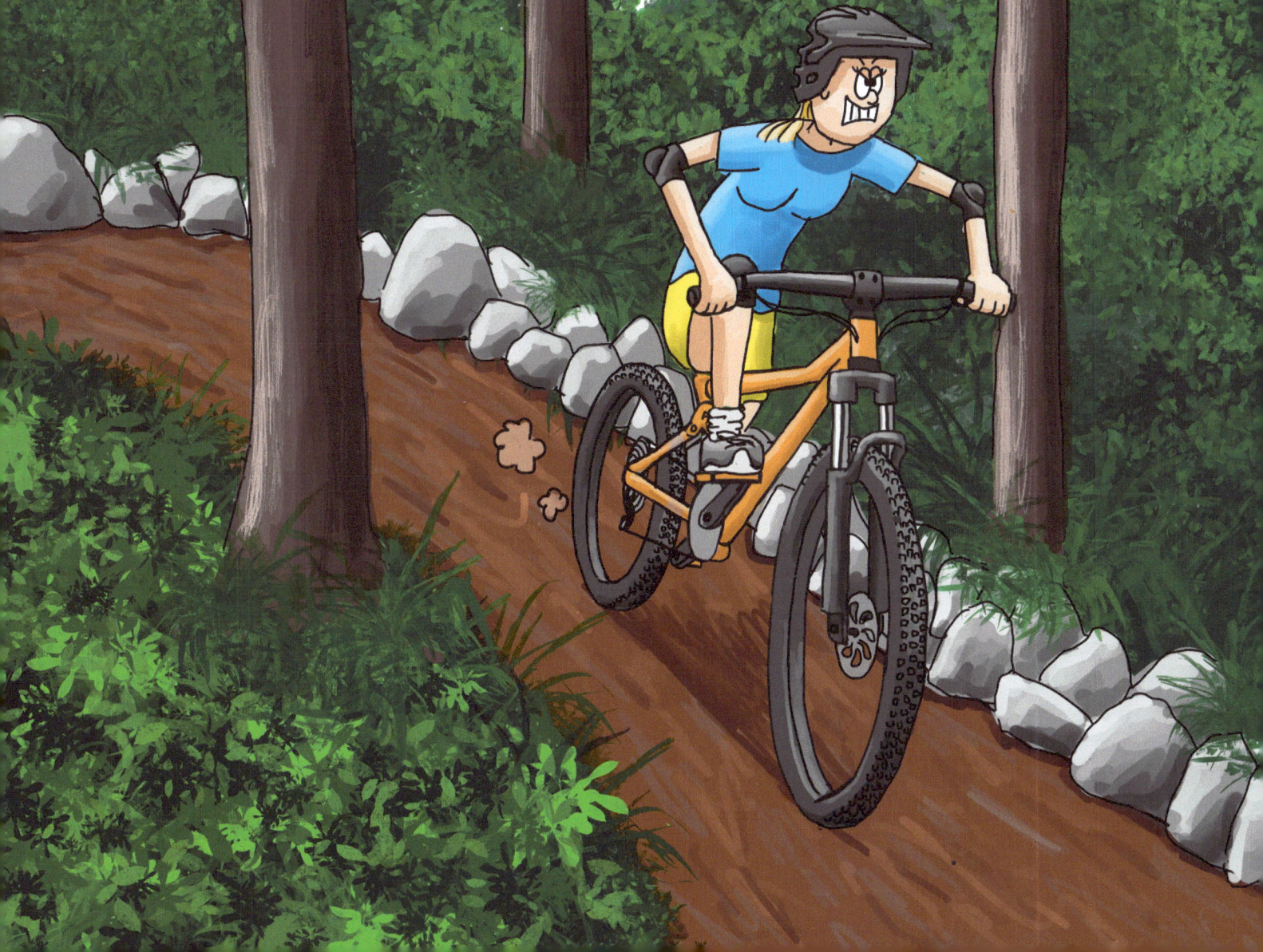

As Dad crossed the line,
Mum was having a snack.

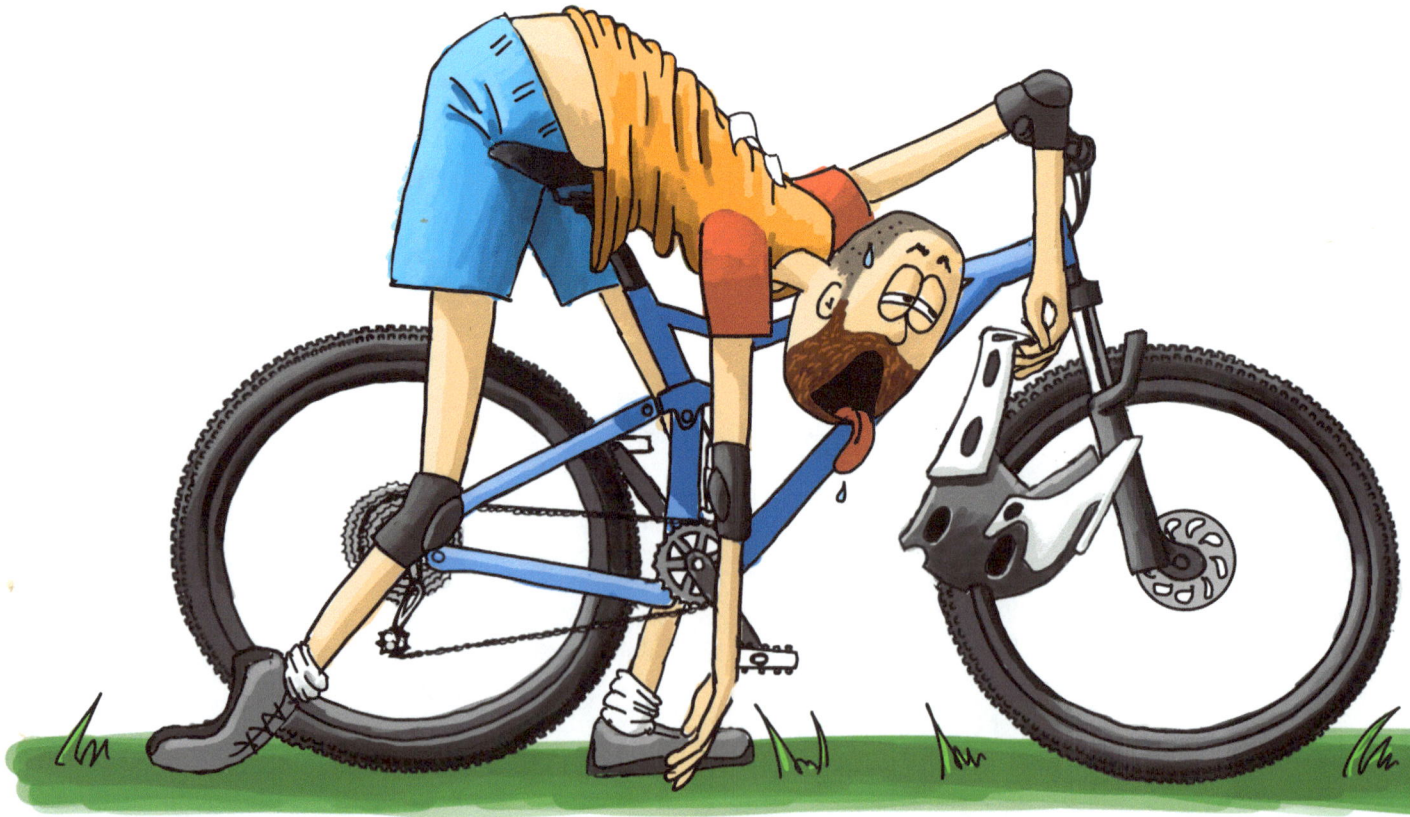

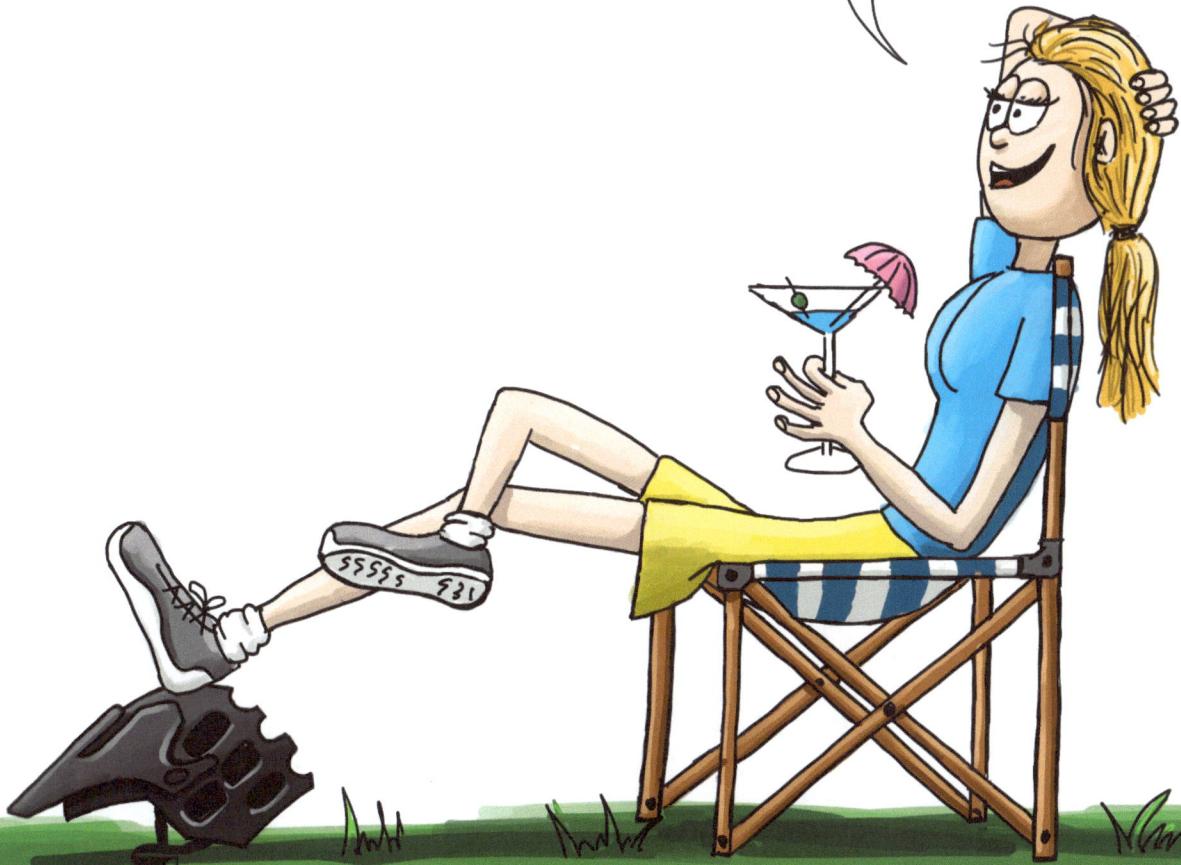

Dad sat in the car,
hands over his head,
and sobbed very quietly
until mum came and said...

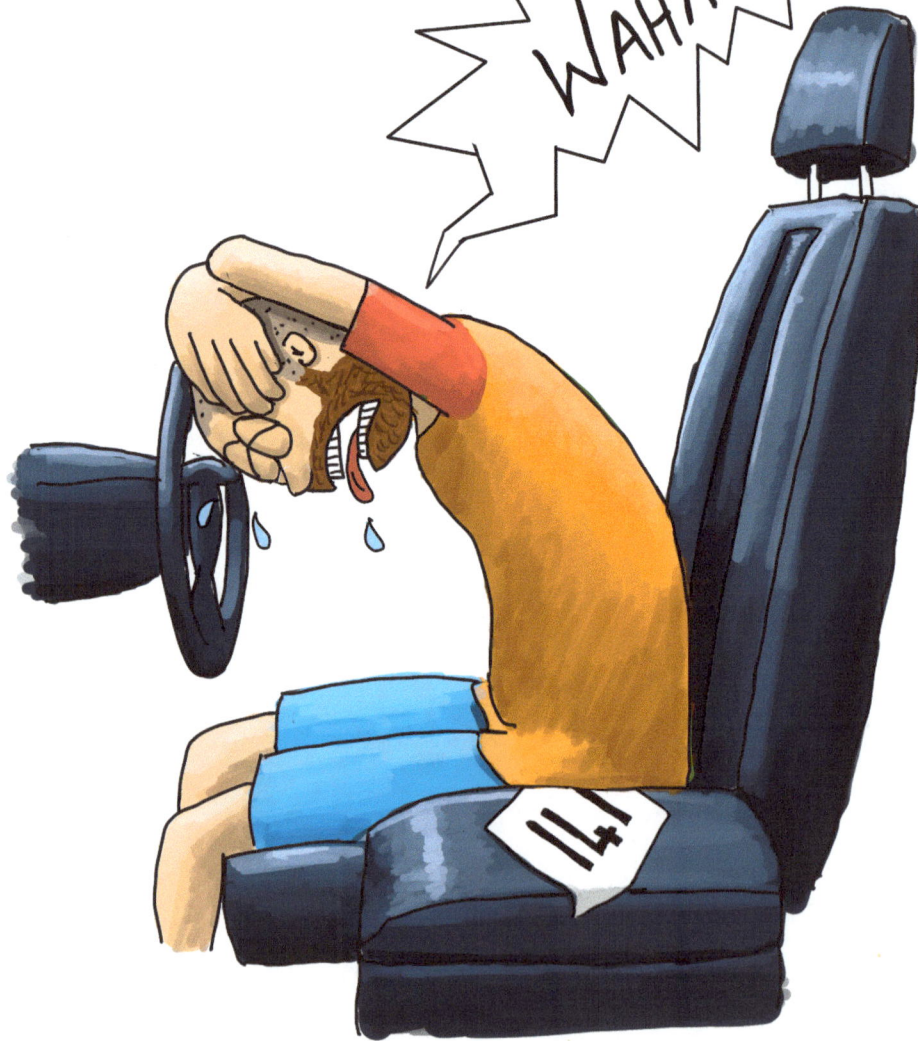

WAHAHAAAA!

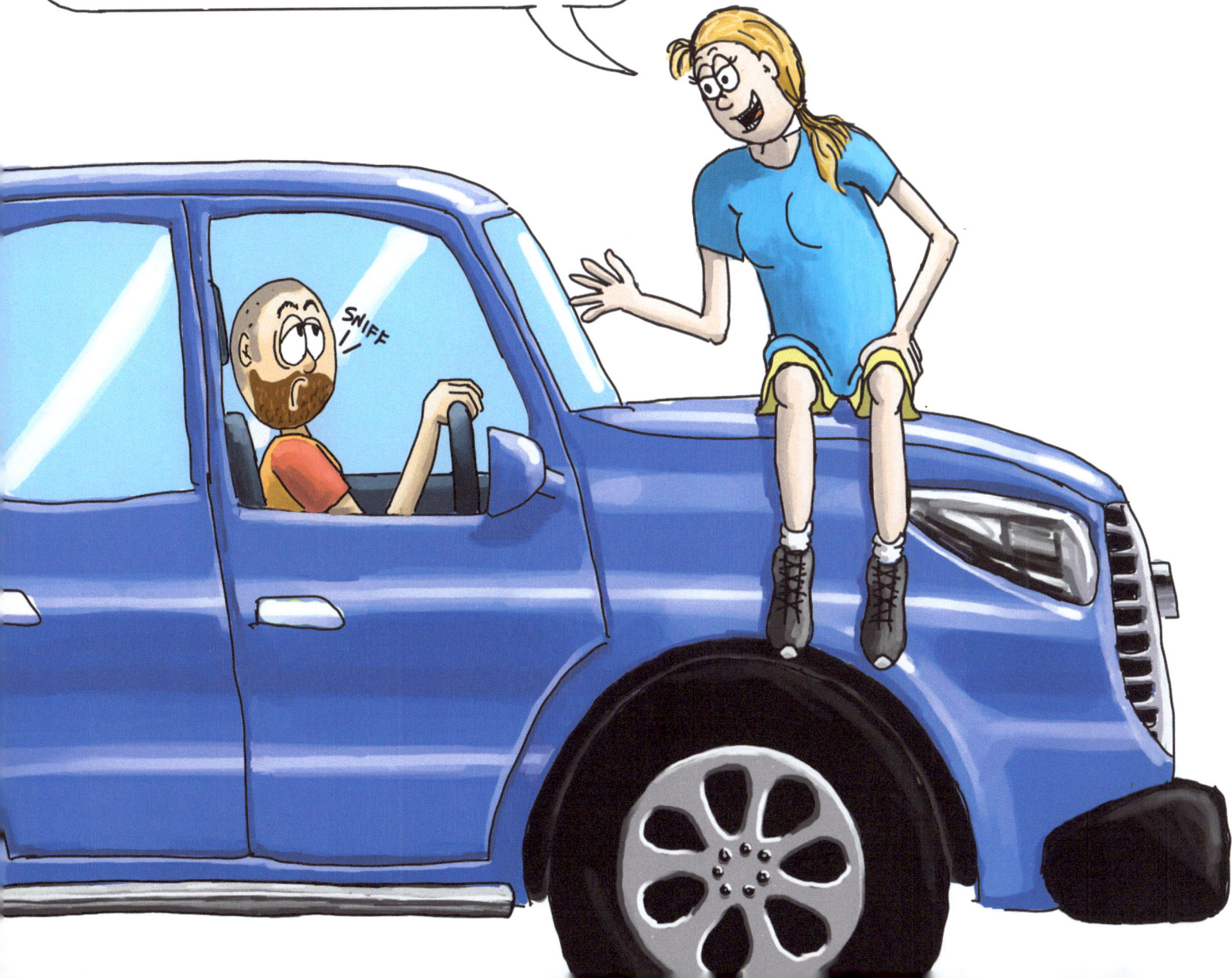

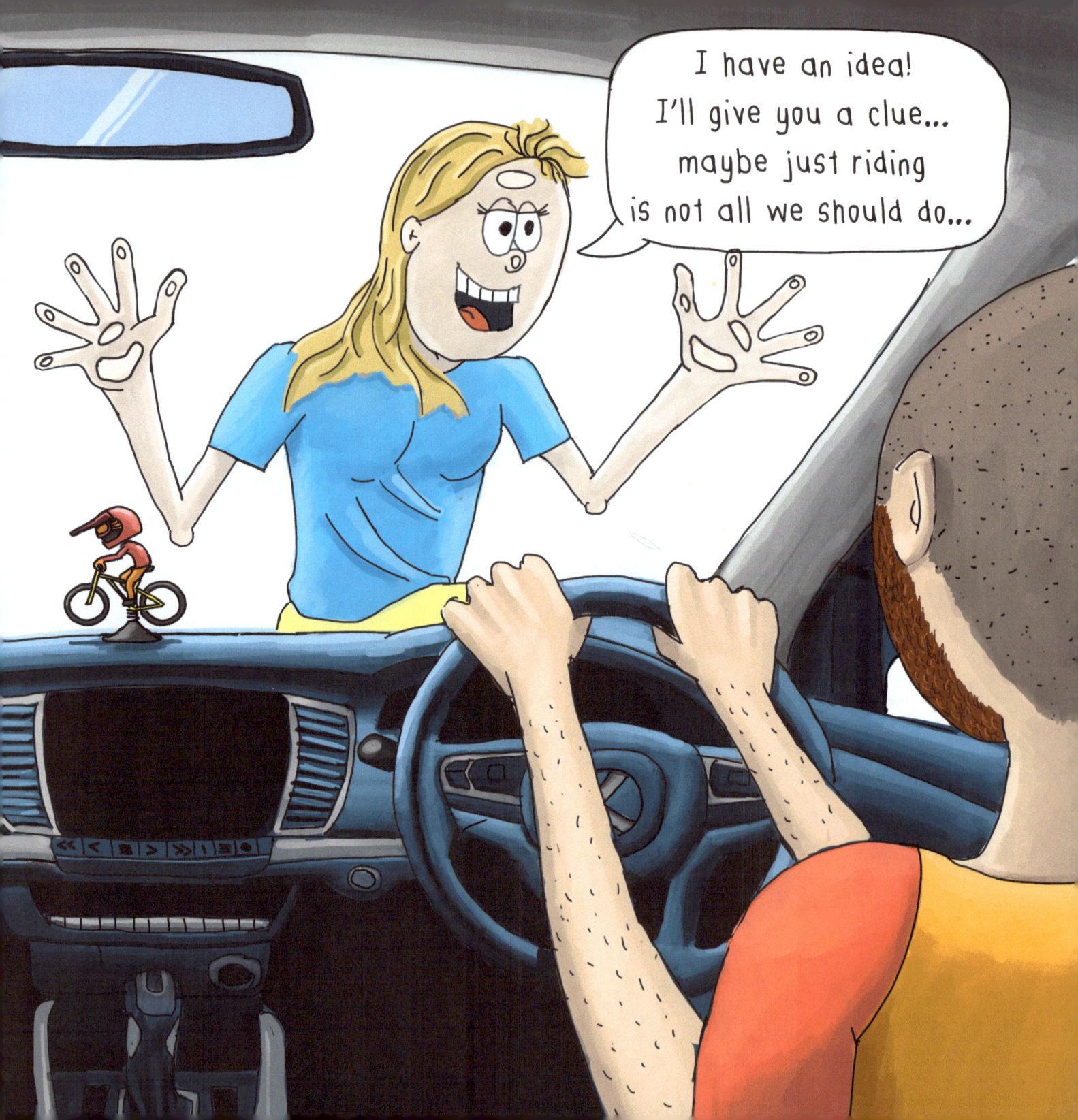

So when Dad finished sulking,
they did something cool.
And started their own...

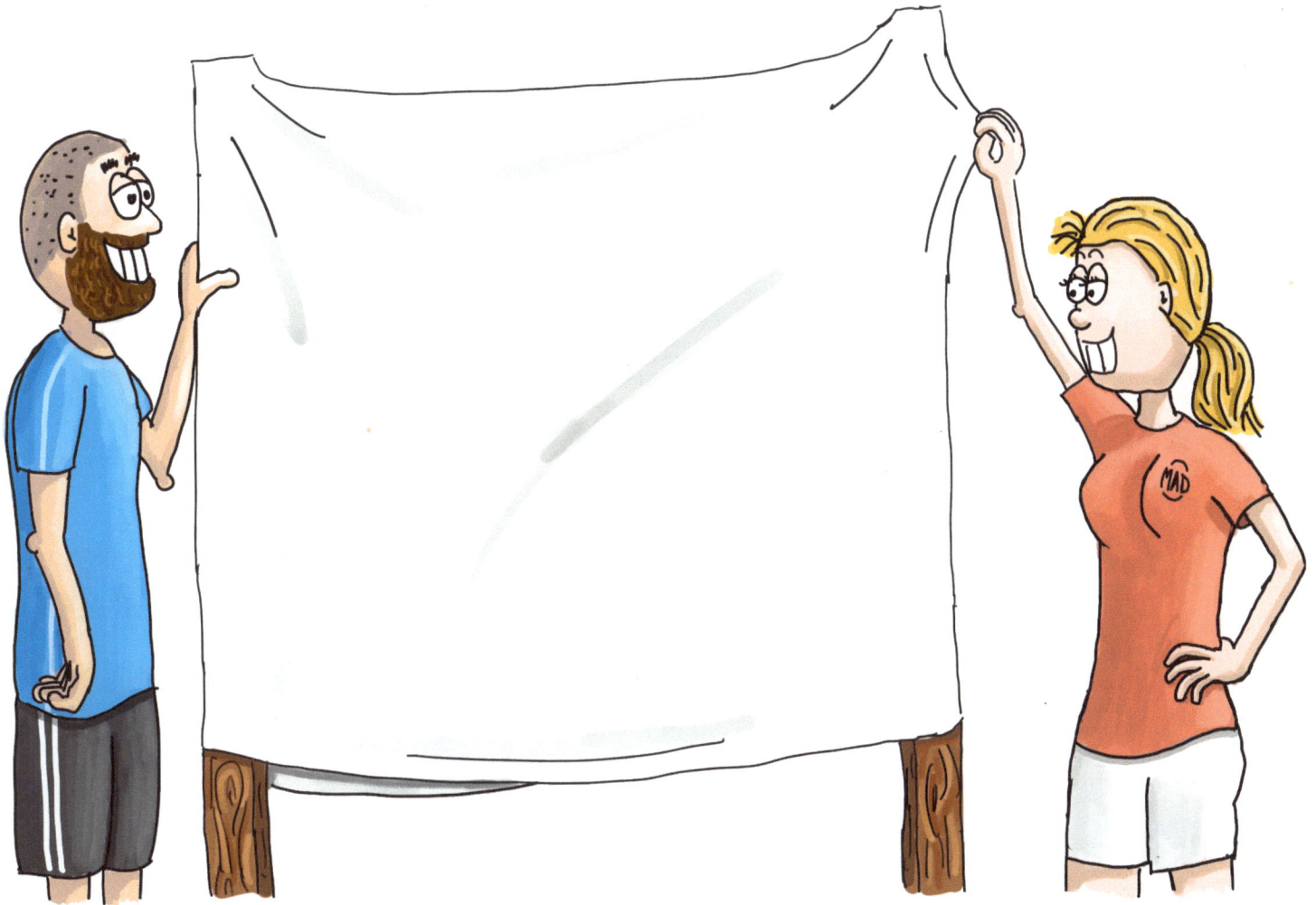

mountain bike riding school!

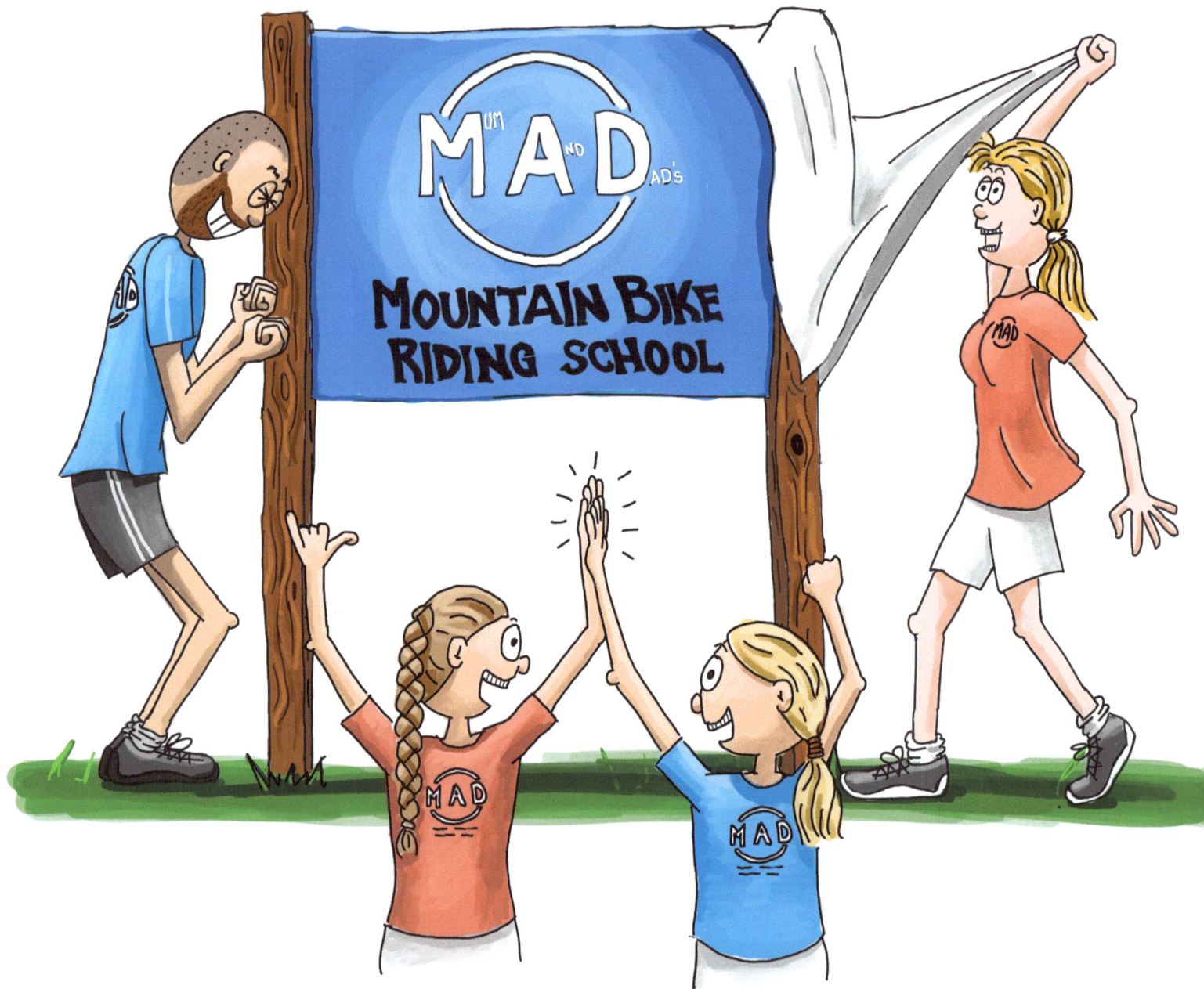

www.ingramcontent.com/pod-product-compliance
Lightning Source LLC
Chambersburg PA
CBHW061138030426
42334CB00004B/92